# NAVIGATING THE JOURNEY OF AGING PARENTS

# NAVIGATING THE JOURNEY OF AGING PARENTS

## WHAT CARE RECEIVERS WANT

### CHERYL A. KUBA

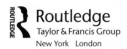

Routledge
Taylor & Francis Group
New York   London

Routledge is an imprint of the
Taylor & Francis Group, an informa business

Published in 2006 by
Routledge
Taylor & Francis Group
270 Madison Avenue
New York, NY 10016

Published in Great Britain by
Routledge
Taylor & Francis Group
2 Park Square
Milton Park, Abingdon
Oxon OX14 4RN

© 2006 by Taylor & Francis Group, LLC
Routledge is an imprint of Taylor & Francis Group

Printed in the United States of America on acid-free paper
10 9 8 7 6 5 4 3 2 1

International Standard Book Number-10: 0-415-95288-3 (Softcover)
International Standard Book Number-13: 978-0-415-95288-0 (Softcover)
Library of Congress Card Number 2005024513

---

### Library of Congress Cataloging-in-Publication Data

---

Kuba, Cheryl A.
    Navigating the journey of aging parents : what care receivers want / Cheryl A. Kuba.
        p. cm.
    Includes bibliographical references (p.    ) and index.
    ISBN 0-415-95288-3 (pb : alk. paper)
    1. Aging parents--Care. 2. Parent and adult child. I. Title.

HQ1063.6.K83 2006
306.874084'6--dc22
                                    2005024513

---

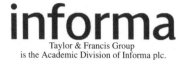

Taylor & Francis Group
is the Academic Division of Informa plc.

Visit the Taylor & Francis Web site at
http://www.taylorandfrancis.com

and the Routledge Web site at
http://www.routledge-ny.com

To my two best guys and girl
Bob, Arthur, and Abby
The true loves of my life

# Contents

# Foreword

Caregiving is a two-way street. I approached the concept of this manuscript as a biased Baby Boomer with membership in a generation whose self-indulgent mantra is, "Hey, what about *my* needs?" Although a portion of this book's audience lived through the Depression era, the majority of readers here represent the Baby Boomer generation, which is hooked on self-help books. My goal was to tell the story of care from the perspective of those who are on the receiving end—the frail, dependent elderly. I did not want to produce a clone of what had been done before—a caregiving book full of opinions *by* caregivers.

At the same time as my parents were taking their own bumpy ride through their last chapters of life—my mom with Alzheimer's disease and dad with poor eyesight and emphysema—I began my search for quality information about families providing care. As a professional in the long-term-care field, I had listened to the experts—the elderly residents of the retirement community where I served as executive director. I wanted to know what kind of care my parents wanted, and I, in turn, would pass on that knowledge to my fellow care providers. Under normal circumstances, I would have asked my mom—except that she was transitioning through the clouded and confusing world of Alzheimer's. During the last year of her life, she was bed bound, and didn't talk.

When I started my personal and professional journeys in researching what care receivers really wanted, I came up short. Each missive and volume I picked up lacked opinions and insights from the care recipients. What started out as a simple report about the void in care-receiver feedback turned into a full-blown thesis for my master's degree in Gerontology.

Nobody, until now, had really listened to the frail elderly regarding care, housing, independence, and dignity because no one had asked the questions. What do they like or dislike about their roles in the caregiving partnership? How do they want to live out the final chapters of their lives? Just as it takes two to tango, it takes two to do the caregiving dance.

We read so many articles, and witness so much about caregiver stress. But, what about *care-receiver* stress? Imagine what the care receiver is facing. He or she must deal with the same dubious, stressful situation as the caregiver, but the care receiver has the added hindrance of dealing with a physical body that is not cooperating.

To get answers to our questions we went to the source—the dependent elderly themselves. A diverse group of receivers were asked their opinions about their own situations, and about independence, love, accommodations, physical care, spirituality, decision-making, and dignity. Our interviewees included farmers, urban dwellers, individuals who had not attended high school, and several who had earned doctorate degrees. Income levels and race diversity were achieved by random sample.

The results are a fact-filled collection of first-person accounts on what it means to be elderly and dependent on a loved one, a friend, or a stranger. The subjects were also very vocal about long-term-care facilities, and the health care workers who run them.

Throughout these pages, care receivers were interviewed about how they feel regarding their current lifestyles. The research revealed that the interviewees want to continue to be very involved in their own care management. Some were angry because they never wanted their elder years to be this way. Many of our interviewees requested that pseudonyms be used instead of their real names. We have respected their wishes.

People are not dependent by choice. It is a mistake to not include dependent persons in every decision. Their opinions matter. Their votes count. Decisions about housing, lifestyle, and care will be made much more easily if the dependent person is involved from the start.

Many snapshots and pieces of life stories featuring the wants and desires of care receivers have emerged in the pages that follow. Some patterns from our interviewees were obvious: many had been caregivers to their own parents; most never thought about old age during their younger years; the majority do not blame a God for their infirmities. Our elderly loved ones want to be heard, have a desire to be involved in their own care, and want to share the wisdom of unconditional love—both while they are dependent and while they are precariously close to death.

The care receivers we talked to held an innate wisdom to problem-solve and get the job done. Prior to her moving into her daughter's three-story townhouse, Anita, 89, had a portable electric elevator chair installed. Brothers Jack and Don problem-solved Don's fall from his wheelchair onto the floor by elevating Don back up to chair seat height through the process of building a makeshift supportive seat with encyclopedias stacked on top of each other. Without this new idea, paramedics would have been needed to get Don off the floor and into his chair. Several members of the early Alzheimer's group who were interviewed here spend tireless days lobbying in front of legislators in Washington to increase funding for Alzheimer's research.

One 89-year-old interviewee showed great remorse in receiving my follow-up thank-you card, because she noticed that it had been manufactured in China. She admonished me for not "buying American." I made a second gesture of thanks to correct my mistake, and sent an American-made thank-you card that had been created by American veterans of foreign wars.

What is quite surprising is that, despite serious illness at this stage in life, only a few of the respondents were unhappy with their lives during this time. Of those individuals who responded, most felt that the best times of their lives was "right now."

If it isn't happiness for the blessings of the moment, then scenes from a healthier, more practical life are remembered. Or, as Ann, 91, asked during our interview, "You want to hear about the best day of my life?' She went on to talk about a particularly bitterly cold winter day in her early twenties when she started out to work at 5:30 A.M. She took three buses to get to her job. Because it was her birthday, Ann decided to play hooky from work, and instead treated herself to a day in downtown Chicago. She went to a movie, Jane Wyman in *The Blue Veil*, and out to lunch. "Then I came home about 4:30, just like I worked. I played hooky the whole day." Although Ann was a world traveler, this was the best day of her life.

It is my hope that this manuscript will not only become a guide to help in your journey with your loved one in his or her final chapters of life, but that it will serve as a reminder of the precious cargo that is within our charge. It is meant to offer hope for family relationships and to renew deeper connections between givers and receivers, whether tied by bloodline, friendship, or compassion.

There are precarious times in our lives when we are each encouraged to "lead, follow, or get out of the way." If you are charged with the care of dependent care receivers, know when to lead on their behalf, recognize how to follow their lead using their opinions and seasoned advice, and be silent and supportive when your own choice might be to run in the other direction.

Every decision we make as caregivers will not be perfect. There will be roadblocks. There will also be smooth sailing. In reading on, absorb what you need and then get behind the wheel with your loved one on board. Enjoy the ride.

# Acknowledgments

It is a humbling experience to have one's name on the cover of a book as the author. This journey could not have taken place without the help and dedication of so many wonderful people. The care recipients who were interviewed, as well as the family members and professionals, are all to be honored as extremely generous people who allowed me to step into their lives. In some cases we talked about sensitive issues, emotional challenges, and difficult family relationships. I am so honored to have had this opportunity. To all who helped me find my way along this road, I offer my most sincere thanks. If I have forgotten to mention your name or omitted a major offering of yours, I regret my error in advance. In whatever way you helped make this book happen, I am grateful.

All of the helpful folks at Routledge Taylor & Francis Group deserve special thanks for making this dream come alive. I am especially grateful to George Zimmar, publishing director, who put his faith in me and guided me through the process. Thank you to Dana Ward Bliss, Brook Cosby, Jay Whitney, Stephanie Pekarsky, and Sylvia Wood for all your support and answers to endless questions.

Victoria 'Tori' Engstrom-Goehry joined me as an interviewer and investigator and I am so fortunate to have her on my team. Her work is professional and her ideas on refashioning some of the material were an added bonus. Thanks to Dani Houchin for showing me the ropes on indexing and other computer technicalities. Helen Schubert deserves special thanks for her lifelong friendship, ideas on promotion, and tips on media contacts. Thanks to Celia Rocks for help with editing early on, Cyndi Maxey and Rita Emmett for guidance on working with agents and publishers, and special thanks to Sue Black for contributing experiences from her former life in hospice work to round out our chapter on death and dying.

Dianne Morr jumped onto this bandwagon months before the writing was finished and rode along with me through editing, rewrites, and proofing. While Dianne's expertise lies in the editing arena, I am so grateful for her personal knowledge of the subject matter, having been a caregiver to her own mother. Dianne offered up wonderful new ideas and different perspectives that have been woven into many of the chapters. Thank you for joining me on this journey.

What a privilege it was to be invited into the unique lives of Les, a Ph.D. professor and former CIA operative; Jenny, a Ph.D. graduate of Oxford University and 30-year health advocate; Sydnee, former flight attendant, gardener, and women's-rights advocate and volunteer; and Cathy, who speaks fluent Italian and was the former chief bacteriologist at the 700-bed Roosevelt Hospital in New York. The common thread that brought us together was their common diagnosis of early Alzheimer's disease. Each person mentioned here allowed me to capture a snapshot of his or her life and gave me a personal assessment of the known and unknown that each expects for the future.

I am especially grateful to Darby Morhardt, MSW, LCSW, and director of education at the Cognitive Neurology and Alzheimer's Disease Center at Northwestern University's Feinberg School of Medicine. She was so helpful to me and to my family when my mother was a participant in Northwestern's Alzheimer's program. Not only did Darby help me with brainstorming for the Alzheimer's chapter in this manuscript, she led me to the Cognitive Neurology and Alzheimer's Disease Center support group, of which the individuals mentioned above were all members.

Peggy Condon was an angel in my life who, as my academic advisor, guided me through my thesis work, and who I had the privilege of getting to know in the deepest sense of friendship during her final days. She honored me by writing the introduction to this manuscript, and my hope is that it will serve as a legacy in her honor.

My fellow sailors from the Catalina Fleet have all contributed a small piece of their lives to this project. Special thanks to Tom and Barb Fitzgerald, John and Lorelei Lauraitis, John and Hazel Luther and Pat and Ron Shereyk for getting their family members involved, and Lorelei Lauraitis and Jim Zagorski for their added perspectives on "only children."

Special thanks go to my spiritual family at St. Paul's United Church of Christ, who willingly volunteered their family members to be interviewed. Betty Barbolini went that extra mile in helping me with an interview during her trip to New York. Sally Kinnamon connected me with several care receivers and professionals to be interviewed. I could count on Marcia Volk as a coach, time management expert, and as a listening ear.

It would take volumes to list all of my friends who have been pillars during this experience. Two need particular mention: Marilyn Granzyk and Kathy Wold. Marilyn's professionalism was a key ingredient in getting the interviews transcribed. As a resource and friend, it was Marilyn who read and reread a lot of my material early on. It was always gratifying to bounce an idea her way or send her part of a chapter at the eleventh hour to say, "Does this work?" No adventure goes unnoticed in Kathy's world, and she is the first to acknowledge an effort with, "I'm proud of you." During the home stretch on the manuscript execution, I received flowers and a note from Kath that read, "Keep that keyboard flyin'."

When this manuscript was still in its idea stage, my best friend Leslie Hughes, and dear neighbors Sid Levin and Natalie Saltiel encouraged me to make it happen and became great sounding boards for various concepts. Some ideas worked, some didn't.

My thanks to all of my extended family, who kept fueling my fire to press on with my work. Ralph Raap deserves plenty of kudos for volunteering to be a wonderful interview subject. Special thanks to Ralph's daughter, Chris Raap, who got me interested in Book Expo, which had the end result of my finding my publisher. Chris also became my personal reference-librarian and willingly answered all my questions no matter how large or insignificant. To my aunts and uncles who contributed many of their own episodes for inclusion in these chapters, I owe a huge amount of gratitude.

Thanks to my sister-in-law Linda, who kept the family gatherings going when I was experiencing crunch time. My sincere thanks to cousins Marian Leben and Nancy Meiki for offering up a play-by-play about their own mother's care, and to Arthur, who consistently reminded me that frequent walks and a gentle nudge could provide a welcome break in a long day at the computer.

So much of what has been written here is a reflection of the journey that my sister Alice and my brother John and I took during the last chapters of our parents' lives. Each decision and each task was made a little easier because we worked as a team. Maybe we are an exception to the norm because we got along, discussed our options, and based our actions on the faith and love of family that Mom and Dad instilled as our foundation. The support and encouragement from John and Alice continue to be such a blessing.

My husband Bob, the center of my universe, has been my co-pilot throughout this wonderful adventure. Where other people in my life have made this book a joy ride, Bob has made it a voyage of fair winds and smooth sailing. In addition to enduring endless nights of take-out food and running the household so that I could keep plugging away, he continually reminds me of the importance of my work. I am fueled by all of his love and emotional support. And, saying that Bob provides technical support is an understatement. What would I have done without him during those numerous times when my computer and printer refused to cooperate?

Finally, I am grateful to God for giving me the resources, talent, and faith to keep going. Through this journey I have enjoyed a spiritual connectedness with so many wonderful people. Blessings to all of you. It's been a wonderful road trip.

## Thanks to the Real Experts

Many men and women, who at the time of this writing were receiving care, shared their innermost thoughts with me about what it means to be dependent on someone else. Several are no longer with us. Many poured out their hearts and souls. We became fast friends. Without the many contributors who were selfless in letting me interview them, this book would not be possible. Thank you from the bottom of my heart to:

| | | |
|---|---|---|
| Dora Alanen | Dorothy Dickert* | Jimmy Lawson |
| Estelle Binder | George Dickert | Anita H. Levin |
| Ella Jean Cleveland | Sylvia Fitzgerald* | Dorothy McClenahan* |
| Floyd Cleveland | Rudy Geary | Steward McClenahan* |
| Dr. Margaret Condon* | George Gifford* | Don Moyer |
| Mary Lynn "Sydnee" | Dan Goldberg | Our friends from Iran |
| Conway | Ann Jerz | Angie Perillo |
| Donald Day | Jenny Knauss, Ph.D. | Ralph Raap |
| John Day, Jr. | Charles Kouba | Ruth Ringstrom |
| Lino Darchun | Loretta Kouba | Rose Schreiner |
| Edward Seely Davis* | Catherine Kraus | Charlotte Seinfeld |
| Barbara Dennis | Herb Kraus | Clifford Yates |
| Leslie E. Dennis, Ph.D. | | Charlotte Zagorski |

*Deceased

# Introduction

Forty Years of Care: My Professor, My Advisor, My Friend

Turning to a master for the definition of life experience in receiving care was my reasoning behind selecting Dr. Margaret Condon to write the introduction. Dr. Condon, "Peggy" was a Ph.D. in Experimental and Theoretical Psychology from Loyola University, as well as a licensed clinical psychologist. She served as my academic advisor for my Master's thesis in Gerontology at Northeastern Illinois University. Through that grueling process, we became good friends. She was the clinical director for the clinically depressed and seriously mentally ill at a residential facility in Illinois and worked in a clinical capacity at the Illinois State Mental Hospital. Having an uncanny affection for dogs and cats, somewhere in Peggy's history she had owned several pet stores, too.

Peggy had first-hand knowledge about being a care receiver. A quadriplegic, she had relied on family, friends, and paid caregivers for her personal care for more than 41 years. As a result of a terrible accident in 1963, when she was 24 years old, Peggy's mobility was limited to use of an electric wheelchair, and she had limited use of her arms and hands. She had relied on the help and support of caregivers—both paid and unpaid—for her activities of daily living, and her everyday tasks since the day of her injury.

Although Peggy had to accept the limitations of her physical being, those limitations only strengthened her resolve. She was chairman of the Psychology Department at Northeastern Illinois University and taught graduate-level classes there for 32 years until her retirement in 2002. Although teaching and mentoring thesis candidates took up the majority of her time, Peggy went on to receive her master's degree in English from

Northeastern the same year she retired. I had the privilege of being Peggy's last thesis student at the twilight of her awesome career.

Her accomplishments were many; her energy was boundless. Her keen sense of understanding regarding the mental processes of human nature—and that of creatures great and small—was beyond comprehension. Peggy died of cancer 12 days after completing the introduction to this book. She was 66. The following introduction is Peggy's personal and professional perspective about "everyday people" becoming dependent on others for care.

**Cheryl A. Kuba**

This is an important book for many reasons, for many groups of people. It's the only book out there that addresses the same issues that caregiver books address, but from an entirely different perspective. This book is timely. There is nothing I have found that directly addresses the perceptions and oftentimes unspoken responses people have to being the objects of caregiving. Everything you read is on how to be a good caregiver, the qualities of a good caregiver, or recently, the need for caregivers to care for themselves.

I'd like to see caregivers get a little insight into how hard it is sometimes to be so dependent on others, and what that feels like from the inside. For care recipients, I know that it would give them some ideas on how to make it a little easier and not feel so totally vulnerable. I would also hope that this book will be read by people who are in neither situation *yet*, of caregiver or care receiver, so that they can be better prepared in one direction or another for what is inevitably going to happen.

I firmly believe that Cheryl's book is appropriate for at least four groups of people. The professional caregivers, who oftentimes don't realize how the small things they do impact the person they are treating; the family caregivers themselves, who are non-professionals, who have only their side of caregiving to look at. The third group is the general public, who has to be reminded often that "care"-giving is often different from caregiving. This book should also be read by health care professionals, who tend to lose sight of the psychological and emotional needs of both groups.

With respect to the first group, the professionals: they are, in many cases, understaffed and overworked. But often, too, overworked and underpaid. They see their job as a job, and their life is their real life. So, consequently, in too many instances they approach people with multiple needs as people who "mess up their schedule" because they have been assigned "X" number of things to do. If you are the person, or care recipient, who ends up taking them longer to tend to, nobody who supervises them allows for that. So, they end up either not doing things people need, or doing them in a hurried fashion. Their actions silently blast, "This is more than what I am supposed to have to do."

My latest experience at a hospital was in December of 2004. I ended up at Loyola University Medical Center, in Maywood, IL. Now, granted, for the first two nights I was on the ICU, where the nurses were given much smaller caseloads and take care of their own patients. They don't just delegate work to nurse's aides and then go off to sit and write or pass pills. It was a wonderful experience because two things seem to have happened. First, the staff who were working with me actually cared about whether I felt good or not in whatever they did for me. The second, which was almost as enjoyable, was the fact that they all worked together. Oftentimes in a hospital, if I needed something that required two people, I would wait a good half an hour before my caregiver could get someone to come in and help them, and that person often came grudgingly.

On this unit, if someone working with me needed a second person, she would stick her head out of the curtain and say, "Can I get some help?" and three seconds later someone else would be there. One morning, as my nurse was finishing up with me, another nurse poked her head in and said, "I'm all done, and is there anything else I can do for you?" The nurse attending to me answered, "I finished everything except this one inventory, but I have plenty of time. Don't worry." But the other gal responded, "Oh, no problem. I've got time, I'll do it."

I then was transferred to the regular floor, and even though I didn't get as much attention on a regular floor as in the ICU (I didn't want to leave), the people who came in to do what they had to do did it cheerfully. Even the graveyard staffs, who are notorious for not doing things the way they are supposed to, were terrific. I required the two-hour body-shift program. One night, the night staff neglected to come. My godchild was staying with me that night. She went and got somebody. They came in and did it. They still came in talking nicely. They didn't feel like someone had interrupted them. It was just nice to have them be pleasant.

I had a visitor who would come often. When a staff member walked in and said, "Hello, how are you?" my friend said, "I think that down at the door where the employees come in, they hand them a cup with a happy pill in it. I haven't met a person in this hospital, that hasn't been pleasant, ready to smile." They are just ready to be friendly. All of a sudden I realized hospitals could be decent places. But, one has to be very careful. I guess Loyola's motto of "We Heal the Spirit" is taken to heart. I'm not saying that Loyola is a perfect hospital, but it was 100 percent better than any other one I have been in.

People tend, if they do a job for a long time, to start leaving off little things that they did at the very beginning. And, up to a point, you just have to put up with it. If you have integrity and dependability in a caregiver, you're 90 percent ahead of the game, so it's worth having to remind people about things. There are also people who do whatever job there is to do, and there are others who form an attachment, and their whole approach to doing the job is different. I think both recipients and caregivers are whatever they are, only exaggerated in their new roles. The care recipient still has the same personality quirks, only is now dependent, and the caregiver wants to go about her day as usual, except she is now in demand.

Another thing I do is always try to appreciate out loud when people do things. It's amazing how, by using "Please" and "Thank You" when either asking for something, or having just received it, really makes a difference in both the care you get and the way the person feels about doing it. Be careful, be appreciative, and try not to lose your patience if things don't go right, because that can only make matters worse. Suppressing yourself, in the long run, pays off.

What I think is important about this book for family caregivers is, even more so than with professional caregivers, recipients are less apt to complain or to try to change how people do things because they are so grateful.

Family caregivers have a hard time because they did not want this to happen to the person they are taking care of, so they are already angry at the universe. They never expected to be in this position, which, in some way, totally disrupts their whole perception of the caregiver's own life. It's very important for them to keep in mind that those are all legitimate feelings, but the place to get rid of them is somewhere other than where you are doing the caregiving.

The secret for me has been to try to make sure that my family knows how to do what needs to be done … but I use them only in emergency situations. This is my first demand. Therefore, I separate my care from my friendships and my relationships. I think that works very well, and I would absolutely recommend it.

Remember, for the family caregiver, the recipient is in a very ambivalent position. On the one hand, it feels comfortable to have someone you know right there. On the other hand, it just floods them with all kinds of feelings of, "This shouldn't be the way it is between us. Who are you? Are you my wife, or are you my nurse? Are you my husband, or are you my nurse?" This ambivalence makes them oftentimes, not only angry at the universe, but angry at you. The recipients don't want you to be the caregiver, but they like you to be that person. So at some times you'll get gratefulness, and at other times more than antagonism, either withdrawal or demands.

Those are the times, even if you can't afford it full time, to bring in a respite person, when you have a space of time so that the family member is not a caregiver.

Often, family caregivers go into the role for the most loving reasons, and it's going to screw up the relationship. You can't be both things at the same time. So the advice is to get as much outside help as you can.

Be there to be the moderator. Be there to be the trainer. Be there to do the inspections and things like that to make sure everything is going okay, but have someone else do the caregiving.

If you cannot get outside help, develop a system. If there is more than one child, create a schedule that makes each one responsible for either only certain days or only certain things. Each person can agree to be the driver all the time, or agree to be the grocery shopper. If they have different days that they are busy, each one feels like they have some sort of freedom. Here are some rules of thumb:

Do a lot of research on things that will make the care recipient feel independent. For example, now there is an electric jar opener. You just position the jar, press a button, and it opens the jar automatically. To do this you have to look, not just in the medical supply catalogues, but in the mail order catalogues—Harriet Carter®, Lillian Vernon®. Very often, you find things there that may be meant for convenience, or for a different reason; but if you look at it for someone who is dependent, you think, "Oh, that will work."

Look for as many ways as possible to make life easier: remote-control buttons, lifesaver buttons, and even remote switches on lamps.

Things happen and you always have to have a back-up plan. If the person you are caring for has no means and no money, there are agencies to turn to: Little Brothers of the Poor; Lions; Rotary; Shriners; Chicago Aging & Disability. There are agencies through the Older Americans Act. People donate stuff. Agencies will redistribute the donated items.

Besides separating my care from my relationships, my second rule is to demand honesty and integrity from caregivers. These people are in my house, all over my house, and have a key to my house. If I feel the least twinge of "I don't think I can trust these persons with all my belongings," I can't hire them.

Because of these two rules, I always try to pay the caregiver well compared with what they would earn in a salaried job. I pay them on payroll so they get social security credit. I realize that I'm speaking from a vantage point that many people don't have, which is one of earning enough money to be able to pay people more than minimum wage. I was fortunate to pay people a rate that was at least five or six dollars above minimum wage.

Otherwise, they can walk from this job to the next and it won't make much difference. For someone like me it makes a great difference because the caregiver is hired for only a half-day, not a whole day. In order for them to be able to make a living, at times I had to adjust my schedule so they could go to another job. It also makes people stay longer if they know they can't get that hourly wage anywhere else. So, often you get people who work a shift that allows them to come when you need them.

I tend, for the most part, to keep caregivers for two, three, and four years at a time, which also makes it much easier. Once they get the routine down, I don't have to monitor the whole process as it's going on. Try as best you can to find a good person or two. Then, when they have to leave, if they are honest and dependable, they may be able to help you find someone they know who meets your criteria. It just begins the chain. I haven't dealt with an agency person in the last 30 years. All of my people have been referrals from other caregivers, or from friends who know caregivers from other jobs, or other contacts they have.

For overnights shifts, I offered room and board in an apartment building I owned. I realize many people can't do this, but I could give the apartment rent-free. The caregiver could do supper, put me to bed, and answer any kind of emergency call I would have during the night.

Now, on to the health care professionals and why this book is so important to them. Health care professionals, in their own way, are caregivers too. The difference is that they often put up a wall where they don't want to know how the care is dispensed really, because they often have too many people to care *for*. They are afraid that, if they also had to care *about*, it would be too much.

Probably my biggest hurdle in the last 41 years has been about perfection. Since I'm a control freak, it is mostly anxiety about, "Is everything being done right?" A long time ago, I mentally separated my body from my person. So even if people were sticking fingers up my bottom, and bathing and moving parts that, in our culture at least, are not the things that other people look at, I could divorce it all. I could say, "This is a mechanism that I have to work in. To that extent, I can still be me." I think this is hard for recipients to do. A lot of them are young, and their self-concept is tied up in their body. I often feel that's how a lot of depression comes about.

The answer to me for that was, when I was in rehab, I had been in graduate school with a group of eight to ten people. They all continued to visit very often. In those visits, they continued to talk about things going on at school, like research. These things made me feel like, "Yeah there are all these physical things going on with me, but they could still talk to me."

Once I could do that, I could just say, "This part, quadriplegic, is just another interference that I have to figure out a way to get around." I would find ways, invent things, and create systems that would allow me to be as independent as possible and to actually be able to be alone.

There are times when I just need to be by myself and still be able to do something like change the channel on the television, turn a page of a book, or type on the keyboard. For me, the answer to that was an excellent occupational therapy program at Northwestern's Rehab Institute of Chicago (RIC). Later, I found Michael, (my handyman from 1973), who always seemed to be able to picture what I pictured. I could say, "I want to do this. I think if we do X, Y, and Z, I think we can actually do it." He could find a way to make it work. Each time I came up with something I couldn't do, I would think about what would have to happen for me to accomplish it. Then I would set about trying to find ways to get it done.

Another answer was to read every disability magazine that was published. I read them all. Often I would find my solution to the problem in the letters to the editor. People would write in and say, "I found this, and it works better." I found an electric (catheter) bag opener there that works every time.

Now that my cancer prognosis has me as terminal, for the most part, people are not treating me differently. Most of my basic bodily care is still being done the way it always was. We'll see, because we won't know where that progresses.

My friends are doing a lot more of the things I used to do for myself, like putting the oxygen in when someone comes, or setting up my computer or my book. They know they don't have to .... It's different from being a caregiver, for example, with someone who has Alzheimer's, where you know it can only get worse, and there can only be more demands on you.

Sometimes when I don't have enough strength in my arms, someone has to feed me. I never had that before. That's a little awkward. But I've gotten used to it. It feels like something okay to do. It's not been a burden; now it's a gift.

**Margaret Condon, Ph.D.**

# CHAPTER 1

# Care Receivers: An Intimate Profile

## The Care Receivers: Knowing Who They Really Are

*"It's a very peculiar sensation. It is horrible. I detest this age! I fight it continually. I can't stand to be this old. Mentally, I would say I'm about 70."*

—Charlotte, 91

Today's elderly who are being taken care of by a family member or by paid help are part of an elite club of 22.4 million individuals (21% of U.S. households) receiving care in the United States. Take a look in your own neighborhood. That means one in four households has someone at home requiring help. The care receivers who are over 85 years of age are part of the fastest-growing segment of the population. Half of them need some help with personal care.

Most care recipients are female (65%) and many are widowed (42%). More than half (53%) live alone. Nearly eight in ten care recipients are age 50 or older. The average age of care receivers over the age of 50 is 75.

In the next few pages, you'll be presented with a vivid and very personal snapshot of the 10 million people in this country who are dependent and elderly and receiving some form of care. In this and the following chapters, you'll hear from the frail elderly themselves about what it means to give up independence. They offer a wealth of information and many possess a trouble-shooting genius that could hold the key to their care, if only they were asked for input. Their life experiences alone are invaluable. They have been central characters of the Depression era; some were alive and active during two world wars. Many of those interviewed here as care receivers

1

have also been in the caregiving role for an elderly relative earlier in their lives.

> *We didn't have any money in those days. We lived in a one-bedroom apartment. My parents slept in the dining room on a day bed, and my grandmother and I slept in twin beds in the bedroom. Sometimes, I would wake up, and my grandmother would be bending over me, very close, to see if I was breathing. She was a wonderful woman. She lived with us until she was 88.*

**—Anita, 89, who lives with her daughter and son-in-law**

Although now dependent, some of these individuals make up for their losses with an innate ability to expose survival tactics as their independence dwindles away. Others see only a dim future. What kind of financial future can care receivers anticipate? What familial relationships are compromised in this intricate dyad of care receiver and caregiver?

> *This disease isn't the worst thing that has ever happened to me. Heavens, no. When I was a young girl in England during World War II we lived across from a bomb dump. You couldn't sleep in the house. We slept under tables made of iron. There were bomb craters all around our house. It was terrifying.*

**—Jenny, 68, diagnosed with Alzheimer's disease in 2002**

### Diseases of the Elderly

As older people live longer, health problems become prevalent and more complex. Often, diseases that result in death will first cause disability and loss of independence for the older adult. The most common causes of death in the United States are cardiovascular disease and stroke. Cancer is the second most common cause of death, followed by diabetes, affecting an estimated 17 million Americans. Diabetes can trigger the onset of stroke, blindness and possibly amputation. While not fatal, arthritis and its painful symptoms affect 60% of individuals over 65 years old.

Dementia, which includes Alzheimer's disease, is most prevalent in people over age 85. Much of the information that exists for caregivers focuses on care for people diagnosed with dementia. While there is information for individuals caring for older people suffering from diseases other than dementia, memory loss and dementia care are at the forefront of the literature.

*The stress of family caregiving for persons with dementia has been shown to impact the caregivers' immune systems for up to 3 years after caregiving ends, thus increasing their chances of developing a chronic illness themselves.*

—(Glaser, J-K. and Glaser, R., 2003)

As our care receivers and caregivers transition together through this journey in the following chapters, you will witness how the "rules of the road" and the complexities of caregiving become less clear regarding family relationships, responsibilities, and the understanding of definitive roles. The emotional ride that both entities encounter includes guilt, remorse, blessings, and adversities turned into opportunities.

In this chapter, you will get a clear understanding about the financial aspects of caregiving, and the $257 billion in free service hours provided by family caregivers. The facts and meaning behind the myth that Americans abandon their elderly is another venue open for discussion. In reality, in the majority of circumstances, the American family is still the number-one caretaker of its older adults. In all, eight out of ten men and six out of ten women live in family settings.

## Who Are Today's Elderly?

Our grandparents and parents, born during the great Depression, are today's frail elders. Many have lived through seven wars and fought in or lived through World War I and World War II. For some who served in the military during the major wars, that experience was their first time away from home in a foreign land. At the time of the World Wars, their generation didn't have the modern-day luxury of television or CNN to bring the battles live into the living room.

When the World Trade Center tragedy happened on September 11, 2001, we were glued to our TV sets. In contrast, when Pearl Harbor was bombed in 1941, our parents and grandparents first heard it on the radio, then took a *World Atlas* off the bookshelf to locate Hawaii … and Pearl Harbor.

The generation that reached adulthood before and during World War II grew up at a time when food was packaged in cans and bottles, and everything from milk to brushes and ice was delivered to one's door. There were no supermarkets or super-sizes. An ice cream cone cost a nickel. There were no video games. There was no shopping on Sundays. Social recreation was probably a Sunday-afternoon walk in the park, visiting relatives, or hours spent configuring pieces into a jigsaw puzzle set up on a card table.

Our frail elderly of today were not part of a "throw-away" society. They saved S&H Green Stamps™ to redeem for household items. They collected bottle caps and saved tin foil. Our elders saw the first airplanes fly and witnessed the birth of both Medicare and Social Security.

Life expectancy for both genders in 1940 was 62.9 years. The majority of care receivers who are featured in this book, were asked about their thoughts regarding old age when they were much younger. Specifically, we asked them how, as young adults, they perceived their lives would play out at this age. Almost unanimously, none of our care receivers gave this stage of their lives much thought when they were younger.

*Did I think about how my life would be at this age? One answer —dead. I thought I would have been killed by a jealous husband by now.*

—Jimmy, 84, happily married 44 years

### The New Tier of Financially Strapped Dependent Elderly

*Paying the Ultimate Price for Healthcare*

According to financial futurists, the reality of a cost-effective plan for receiving health care has come to this: You need to be really rich or really poor to cover your health care costs in the United States. The majority of individuals who are our nation's elderly middle class are surviving on pensions, fixed incomes, personal savings, and social security. Many fall into the category of being uninsured or underinsured and are feeling the financial pinch of escalating health care costs. Even for the insured, rising costs of prescription drugs and out-of-pocket health care costs are overwhelming older adults who find their financial resources stretched to the limit.

*Last year turned out to be a really expensive year for me. After my wife's stay at the nursing home, paying the caregiver, my surgery, and all of our medications for our various ailments, I ended up spending about $25,000 out of pocket for our health care. That's after what Medicare paid for. And I always thought we had good insurance.*

—George, 89

Although the 2005 federal poverty guidelines released February 18, 2005 raised the basic poverty figure to $9,570 for an individual, an increase of $260, that increase doesn't make a difference to the elderly middle class. Seniors who have too much income to qualify for Medicaid, but are just above the poverty line, fall through the reimbursement cracks. As a result of escalating heath care costs, these individuals are forced to choose between getting prescriptions filled or paying the mortgage and household bills.

Seniors spend more, both in real terms and as a percentage of their incomes, on health care than other segments of the population. In 2002, older consumers averaged $3,586 in out-of-pocket health care expenditures, an increase of 45% since 1992. In contrast, the total population spent considerably less, averaging $2,350 in out-of-pocket costs. Older Americans spent 12.8% of their total expenditures on health, more than twice the proportion spent by all consumers (5.8%). Health costs incurred on average by older consumers in 2001 consisted of $1,886 (53%) for insurance, $955 (27%) for drugs, $582 (16%) for medical services, and $163 (5%) for medical supplies.

In 2003, adults aged 65 and older in the U.S. filled an average of 26 prescriptions per year. The high was 37 prescriptions in Tennessee, compared with a low of 16 prescriptions in Alaska. Prescription prices differed depending on the state where the elder lives. The average price per retail prescription varied from $45 in New Mexico and Arkansas to $67 in Alaska and the District of Columbia. The figure includes retail prescriptions filled per capita, the average price of prescriptions, and total spending on retail prescriptions in each state.

Medicare pays for slightly more than half (54%) of the overall health care costs of its enrollees age 65 and over. This population pays 21% of their health care costs out of pocket. Medicaid covers 10% of costs, and private insurers, as well as other payers, primarily cover another 15%.

> *I had planned to leave money to my brother, but my care is eating all of that up. Now I am having to cut into my principal.*
>
> **—George, 77, diagnosed with ALS and paying a full-time caregiver**

By 2006, the average family health insurance premium will exceed $14,500; premium costs will have increased by more than $5,000 in just 3 years according to a report by the National Coalition on Health Care, (May 2003.) In a similar report released by Families USA (McClosky, 2000) the national organization for health care consumers, average drug bills are projected to more than double in the next 10 years.

Older adults take the largest financial hit when it comes to paying for prescription medications. Seniors make up the largest percentage of consumers who buy prescription drugs. The typical American senior taking three prescription drugs paid $175.56 more for medications over the 12 months ending in September 2004 than over the previous year, according to the most recent figures published from AARP (Gross, D., Raetzman, S., Schondelmeyer, S.W., 2005). Of the 197 drugs most used by elderly patients, 161 went up in price during that time.

> *Consider this: According to Ron Pollack, executive director of Families USA, about the Medicare drug cost information that became law in 2003, by 2006, most seniors will pay an annual premium of $420 for drug coverage. Within a decade, that premium will increase to $816. Simultaneously, the drug deductible will grow from $250 to $472. And, worst of all, the huge gap in coverage in which seniors will have to pay 100% of their drug costs—the so-called "doughnut hole"—will grow from $2,850 to $5,382. It is tragically clear that seniors will find that, under the new Medicare law, the costs of medicines will become increasingly unaffordable.*

## Meet the Caregivers

There are only four kinds of people in the world:

1. Those who are currently caregivers
2. Those who have been caregivers
3. Those who will be caregivers
4. Those who will need caregivers

—**Roslyn Carter (1997)**

Who is providing the care? We are: those of us who are spouses, daughters, sons, grandchildren, cousins, nieces, and nephews. Family caregivers provide approximately 80% of homecare services. Becoming a family caregiver can come with its burdens and rewards. The *caregivers* who are family members struggle in their duties with emotional issues of guilt, role reversal, family issues, and their own personal health. In some instances, the relationship between the family member providing care and the older adult becomes enriched. No two cases are the same. The rapport among siblings, adult children, and their elders, once estranged, has often been strengthened through this journey.

People who rise to the task of lending a hand or putting their own lives on hold to work for a loved one day and night are a special breed. Sometimes called "informal caregivers," these individuals provide unpaid assistance to elderly loved ones. Research studies estimate that there are 44.4 million American caregivers (21% of the adult population) age 18 and older who provide unpaid care to an adult age 18 or older. These caregivers are present in an estimated 22.9 million households

(21% of U.S. households). On average, an individual will serve as a caregiver for 4.3 years.

## The Generation of Caregivers

The adult child, the "baby boomer" born between 1942 and 1963, was part of the generation that saw the evolution of television: first in black and white and then in color. Our first action heroes that came to life through television were Daniel Boone, Superman and Marshall Dillon of Gunsmoke. The closest contact the baby boomers had with reality TV during their formative years was through the fictional characters of Moe, Larry, Curly and the Mouseketeers.

With the technological communication explosion creating super cyber highways through the Internet, cable TV, and interactive video, today's baby boomers have been jettisoned into a new reality, one where up-to-the minute information can be accessed with a click of a button. As the baby boomers grow older, they are becoming savvy consumers who can gather resources without leaving the comfort of their homes. They can also choose to be very discriminating in all areas of their lives, including finances, entertainment, and the vast, and often confusing world of health care.

More than 70 million baby boomers will retire by the year 2008. Many of these retirees are still taking care of an elderly relative. Since Americans are living longer, it isn't unusual for a 70-year-old retired man who is both a grandfather and father, to have the responsibility of managing care for a 90-year-old mother or father. Here's an interesting statistic: If you are a woman who has reached age 50 with no occurrences of cancer and no heart disease, your life expectancy can be 92.

### The Caregivers: When It's All in the Family

The typical family caregiver is a baby-boomer woman in her mid-forties. She's employed and spends about 18 hours a week taking care of a parent in his or her late 70s, usually her mother. Although the spouses and partners of the dependent elderly are rarely the targeted market for caregiving information, spouses make up 48% of the caregiving population in this country. Many siblings of the frail elderly are also providing care.

Another dimension of the typical caregiver's world is her role in the sandwich generation—a man or woman who has children still living at home, and also has the responsibility of taking care of an aging parent. An even more complex family component that has revealed itself as the general population lives longer is the multi-tiered sandwich generation. This segment, the double-tiered sandwich generation, is composed of adult children who are grandparents themselves, yet are continuing to care for their own parents. It is not unusual to have four and even five generations exist in a family as people continue to live longer.

> *I'll tell you, when my husband died, Pat, my daughter, said to me, "You take care of yourself as long as you're able and when you're not able to take care anymore, I'll take care of you." That's what she told me at the funeral home. I lived alone for 11 years. When I got sick, I got sick in the middle of the night, when they were out of the city, out of the state. Twice that happened to me. So I started to think, well, what if this happens and I'm alone and I'm not able to get to the phone, and all that stuff. I was tired of being alone. That's what it was.*

> —Angie, 86

Angie, and her daughter, Pat, sold their respective homes to buy a larger house and live together. Angie has lived with her daughter, son-in law, granddaughter, and two cats for more than 4 years.

The portrait of the "typical" caregiver becomes quite blurred when you consider that more men are becoming involved in care. Men now make up 44% of the caregiving population according to the National Family Caregivers Association (NFCA) *Random Sample Survey of 1000 Adults* (2000).

Some men willingly volunteer to provide care for their aging dependent spouse or parent. Others do so grudgingly, against their wishes, and without choices or options. In research gathered from focus groups I conducted, caregiving spouses, particularly male caregivers, either felt that they were completely isolated or had no access to resource information about caregiving.

Consider, too, that while most family caregivers are related by blood or by marriage, many common-law partners, colleagues, neighbors, and friends have taken on the role. However, the majority of caregivers, estimated at 80%, are family members.

### Caregivers in the Work Force

More than 14 million U.S. workers care for an aging family member. These workers are either baby boomers, born during the two decades after World War II, who are looking toward their own future; or are Generation Xers, in their 20s or 30s, born to baby boomers. A recent study calculated that American businesses lose between $11 billion and $29 billion each year due to their employees' need to care for loved ones 50 years of age and older. Nationally, about 10% of working caregivers take early retirement or leave corporate America altogether as a result of their caregiving responsibilities.

Due to the strain of absenteeism and drop-out from the work force of employees who leave for caregiving responsibilities, companies have become more focused on elder care. Many companies now include elder-care counseling and resources in employee benefits packages and in the firm's employee assistance programs (EAP).

The dynamics of care providers' work schedule, as well as home life, can be greatly affected by their new responsibilities. At the same time, receivers' needs become a priority depending on their levels of health, fitness, or frailty.

The roles of both care receiver and caregiver are sometimes divisive and complex. The boundaries of familial roles can become diluted when a caring relative is thrust into a decision-making capacity for a family elder. For others, the new connection reveals richness in newfound companionship or a newly discovered path to repaired relationships.

# CHAPTER 2

# Start the Conversation

## Our Elderly Relatives Talk About What They Want

*It's just the fact that they've come to help and I should just sit back and let them help, and not be like I'm not grateful ... and those are the silly decisions I'm talking about. Very silly. I mean my daughters have not been forceful in anything about changing our lifestyle. When I get in the car they buckle me up and they baby me. And I don't like it.*

—Delores*, 82

"Start the conversation." This was one of the sarcastic greetings that my dad would use to answer the phone in his later years. He wanted to be in control of the conversation, and he didn't want to muddle through the standard greetings of "Hello" and "How are you?" He wanted the caller to get to the point. "Start the conversation," was Dad's way of cutting through the clutter.

So much has been written for adult children who are caregivers about how to discuss difficult topics with aging parents. This chapter turns the tide and lets our dependent elderly open up and sound off regarding best practices for *starting the conversation* about the tough stuff—personal finances, declining health, loss of independence.

---

* not her real name

### The Desire to Open Up

Older adults who rely on care from others, especially family members, feel the need to open up to their care providers because of their own past experience with their elders, or with children. Whether they take the next step or remain in their own private domain is another matter.

Anita, 89, who lives with her daughter and son-in-law, reverts back to her early family relationships. "I knew with my own children early on that I had to talk with them about problems. I did get outside help, too. As a young mother I talked to the librarian and asked for any books they had on child psychology. The librarian couldn't have been more helpful. After she gave me the books, she said, 'Come in and we'll discuss them after you read them.'"

Anita was an only child who didn't have a close relationship with her own mother. In turn, her mother had an unusual way of looking at problems with Anita. "When I was growing up, my mother was never a person who would sit down and talk with me. She called in everyone else to see about the problem. She would call in school counselors, neighbors, and friends. But she never talked to me."

### Dual Challenges

More often than not, most elderly individuals would choose to remain fiercely independent, but would accept help when needed. Recognizing that perfect time to offer help, and sometimes having to insist on getting help, is a challenge. Getting parents to discuss their present situation is the way to get the best information about their needs.

A great way to offer assistance is to explain to elders that accepting help in one area of their life may enable them to live more independently in another. For example, if the care recipient is having trouble with dressing and personal hygiene, perhaps bringing in a home-care aid for bathing and dressing will free up the recipient to feel and look better to get out and socialize.

### What's Behind the Resistance?

When my parents lived in a retirement community and my father could no longer drive, he refused to ride on the bus that the community provided. Thinking that money might be his motivator, I explained that the bus service was paid for out of his rent money, and that he should take advantage of this service. When the reason behind his resistance came out, it had nothing to do with who paid for the bus. In my dad's opinion the bus was full of … "too many old people."

If an aging family member is reluctant to use services offered through public assistance or government programs, remind them they have been contributing funds for these services all their working lives through tax dollars and social security.

## Where Do We Begin?

Bringing in a third source, such as a news article about a difficult care situation, can act as a conversation opener. Perhaps one of your parent's friends is having a mobility challenge, or has to move to a long-term care facility. Using something that is familiar as an example is a good way to open communication.

Be prepared. Once the communication has started, don't be surprised if what you wanted to hear doesn't happen. Open communication is a two-way street, and this could be the perfect opportunity for loved ones to campaign for independence. Perhaps they will present a demand to be met. Do your homework. Explore all possibilities in making them safe, and happy.

> *Recognize that you're stepping into the shoes that carried you across—or to the boots that carried you across—the river. And it's the hardest job in the world: to be a parent to a parent.*
>
> —Jimmy, 89

If a one-on-one discussion doesn't seem to work, you can write out your concerns. Setting your thoughts down in a letter is a good approach. Seeing your discussion topics in writing may help your elderly family member read and ponder your suggestions.

## Communicating Through Others

Sometimes you are not the person who your care recipient wants to tell about all of his or her physical or financial concerns. If there is a favorite relative or special adult grandchild, enlist his or her help. Explain to the intermediary that you are not trying to interfere; you just want to open up the lines of communication.

Focus or discussion groups facilitated by senior centers can be another outlet. If your aging relative is able to get out, these groups can offer a wonderful opportunity for discussion with peers of similar age and interest. This exchange of ideas can create an environment where the care receiver feels comfortable to discuss difficult issues. For individuals who are homebound, offer to host a discussion group at their own home—and you can serve as the host or hostess. Let everyone know that you will honor their privacy.

## Better Communication Through Education

Whether it is Alzheimer's or any of the other debilitating diseases that are common to the elderly, it is easier to open up the lines of communication if all parties have access to educational materials on the disease. Family members and friends have different modalities for learning, according to Darby Morehardt, MSW, LCSW, director, Education Cognitive Neurology and Alzheimer's Disease Center at Northwestern's Alzheimer's Disease Center. "Some family members learn about the disease by attending seminars; others ask for pamphlets, and many rely on the knowledge of their doctors. In whatever way they learn, they must absorb as much as possible."

> *The eldest of seven children, Sydnee said that her younger sister, Emily, had the most difficulty with the news of Sydnee's Alzheimer's diagnosis. "She thought that only males got Alzheimer's. I said, 'Emmy, it's a disease that hits everybody. It doesn't make any difference if you are male or female.' And she has been panic-stricken for a long time.*

## Respect

To keep and maintain a sense of harmony, each household member, or friend of an elderly person in need, has to demonstrate respect for the elder in all good works and deeds. Nothing will be accomplished in terms of happiness, harmony, and quality care if respect and dignity are not honored.

When the discussion between a caregiver and a care receiver turns to sensitive issues such as finances, personal health, or relationships, the elderly loved one needs to be reassured that confidentiality will be maintained and that his or her privacy will be respected.

> *About Dignity: The person who treats me with dignity is the person who knows what to do to give me help—as long as they have an open mind about that. When I say open mind, that they are willing to show me or guide me along the way so that I can receive the help with dignity.*
>
> *Well, dignity is just a state of mind based on acceptance of a deed or kindness or exchange with recognition that this is ... done in a manner that would be welcome by both the giver and the receiver.*
>
> —Jimmy, 89

## Communication Across the Generations

With the exception of spousal caregiving, the care dynamics within a family most likely span across two generations, and with grandchildren in the mix, across three. Consider that your elderly loved one grew up in a different time, at a different pace. Airplanes weren't supersonic. Telephones had a rotary dial, and long-distance calls were placed through an operator. Elders' explanations and observations about everyday life need to be understood and respected. Your attitude and acceptance of their opinions is critical.

## Sounding Off on Accepting Help, and the Perfect Care Provider

Individuals who participated in interviews for this book have very definite ideas about care and their expectations about care providers. While many of our interviewees wouldn't share this information with their caregivers, they opened up with their opinions and advice for our readers. Here is what they had to say:

About helpers in a long-term care facility:

> *The caretakers could be more understanding, and not provoked about everything. One will be real nice; the other will be just the opposite. If I didn't know what I know about this place, it would make a difference. Try and talk to them (adult children) and explain it. There's no one that is going to take care of you like they do in a nursing home.*
>
> —Charlotte Z., 94

> *Act as though the situation was reversed, and the (adult child) needed the help, and what they expected me to do. It gets back to the old "do unto others as you would have them do unto you." Treat me as they would want to be treated.*
>
> *Whether they are a nurse, or whatever care they're giving, that they do it with gentleness, kindness, and respect. If I'm the receiver or if I'm just the observer of it, I think it's necessary that there be open communication. Otherwise, it gets them to the point where communication can be awfully awkward.*
>
> —Jimmy, 89

About family caregivers:

> *I would tell children to take care of their parents. Take care of yourself and take care of your parents. To be close to them. Because you never know. Because someday you'll get old, too.*

> —**Ann, 92**

> *I think sometimes when your children come, maybe they're a little more apt to take over. I don't say that reluctantly 'cause I think they're trying to do it to give me a break. But, I am grateful, and they're very good about it. And with three daughters, you know (there are) three different personalities. They all do it differently.*

> *I don't really feel they're taking over. You just think maybe once in a while they'd ask you, "Would you like this done?" instead of going ahead and doing it. But that's just a picky thing. I don't know if I feel bad saying it. When you're a very independent person, it kind of gets to you sometimes.*

> —**Delores, 82**

Worries about being a burden:

> *Well, I want for my daughters and their families to have a good life and not be burdened with worries about us. I mean, that sounds very righteous, but I do. I think they're getting to an age where, you know—a couple of mine are in their 50s—and if they don't start enjoying it and doing some of those things now, it's going to be later than they think. And I don't want to have to feel like they've got to come home and be burdened with our care.*

> *My mother died when she was in her 70s. Some of those years after the girls got older were some wonderful years in our life, too. We were able to do things we never got to do before. And I want them to do that. I really do. I mean, I think that's one of my goals. And even if we go into a nursing home, I'm hoping that we can leave them something. I'm not saying that I'm going to deprive myself of anything, but we were fortunate with his folks and my parents leaving us something and it has made a difference in our lifestyle.*

> —**Delores, 82**

Many of the care receivers interviewed here had been caregivers of aging parents earlier in their lives. Drawing on that former experience has influenced some decisions about their own family relationships and care environments.

Speaking from experience as a former caregiver:

> *Well, (my husband) Fred's mother was real ill for a long time with cancer, and I took care of her. We lived here at that time, and she lived in her own home, but I was able to do a lot for her, which I am grateful for. I took care of her. I took care of my sister-in-law. I took care of my mother. And I was glad that I could do it, and I never resented it. But as I say, I was younger when I did it, too. I just feel that at their age, I don't want my daughters to be saddled with that if I can help it. Because life is short. It goes by pretty fast.*

—Delores, 82

### Action Steps

- Let aging relatives know that discussing concerns about one area of their lives could help give them more independence in other areas as well.
- Bring in a news article that features topics similar to those issues you would like your loved one to discuss.
- Enlist the help of a third party such as a favorite adult grandchild or friend. Let the third party know that there will be no violation of trust or confidentiality.
- Find senior support groups through senior centers or churches. Your family member may open up after meeting with like-minded individuals of a similar age.
- If your care receiver is homebound, offer to host a discussion group at his or her home, and then give the group privacy.

Given time, care receivers may sort out some of their feelings about privacy, sharing personal business details and their willingness to accept help. No matter what the outcome, opening the lines of communication is a critical component in the delivery of care. Delores had second thoughts about her adult daughters' good intentions. "I'm probably too darned independent. I can buckle myself in the car. Those are the little … insignificant, not important things. I probably should sit back and enjoy it. And I should just learn to not bristle and be grateful they want to do it, and I'm going to try harder."

# CHAPTER 3

# Take Care of Yourself First

### Learn How to Enjoy the Ride

The captain has turned off the seat belt sign. You are now free to move about the cabin.

Unfasten your seat belt. Take a walk around. Bask in this sense of calm.

"What calm?" you ask. Aren't you the caregiver whose head is whirling at a million miles an hour? Don't you feel like the juggler on the old "Ed Sullivan Show" who is spinning the dinner plates of life up on balancing sticks?

Whether you are a caregiver, a friend of a caregiver, or a sibling who is trying to figure out how to help, take a break and *pay close attention to this chapter.* By applying the techniques you will learn here, you will be able to calm your fears and control the chaos of caregiving. It will mean the difference between being driven to distraction and enjoying the ride. The choice is yours.

### *When You Are Already in Trouble*

When you read any of the hundreds of brochures about caregiving, or attend any caregiver training seminars, one of the first pieces of advice you'll hear is, "Take care of yourself, before you take care of others." The classic example that follows is usually the one about the safety features on an airplane. *"Secure your own oxygen mask before you help your child with his or her mask."* Blah, blah, blah. Call me flip about this misdirected advice, but by the time you, the caregiver, are instructed to put on your oxygen mask, it's too late. The plane is going down.

You need to get a grip *before* the first sign of turbulence. You can't wait for instructions from the flight attendant. *Get your own oxygen mask on now.*

### Listening To and Hearing What Care Receivers Want

No two situations are alike when it comes to care management. Whether the care plan calls for the family caregiver to provide "hands on" help, or to bring in a paid care provider, the care receiver will have a voice, and genuine concerns about the new arrangements. Many, like Estelle, want to send a clear message to their family members about both positive and negative experiences with caregivers.

> *Estelle, 94, lives in a senior-citizen housing complex on Chicago's north side. She feels very strongly about her most recent caregiver. Here is her story:*
>
> *I wasn't feeling good, and my daughter got this lady because she knew she took care of somebody else that died. So that's the only thing we know about the woman. She's from Honolulu or something and my daughter got her to stay with me. She stayed here all night, too, on the couch, and it was getting quite expensive. I said, "Gee. It's costing me a lot of money for her."*
>
> *My daughter said, "Yeah, but Ma you're sick. What's the use of saving the money? What's the use of saving it?"*
>
> *So [the caregiver] stayed here, and I told her, "If you want to work short hours, O.K." She didn't like that, but then she gave in. Because I felt she was too old herself to be a caretaker, you know. And then she came in from 9 to 3, but at a quarter of three she had to leave because this bus stopped running that would take her to the CTA bus line. She used to grumble about that a lot. I don't know. We just didn't mix, she and I. She'd make breakfast and then dinner. And then she'd say, "Oh, I've got these leftovers from yesterday. You can have that for lunch when I go."*
>
> *I don't think she was any good … she didn't look after me enough, you know. If she had looked after me more, she would have prepared something. But she never did. And she thought, "I can always go back and make more money than I get over here." She would tell me that all the time.*
>
> *So she said she was going to go, she wasn't going to take this stuff any more. She went. I was glad she went, because I couldn't tell her that I didn't want her anymore. I didn't know how to tell her. So, when she says she's going to quit, I was thinking, "Let her do what she wants." She wasn't fit to be a caretaker. I told her, "Well, the only*

*reason that you got along with that other woman was because she died. She wasn't saying anything to you."*

### Driven to Distraction

How do you as a caregiver know when you are driving too close to the edge? At your first sign of executing some task dysfunctionally, stop and reassess what you are doing. When you are lost—physically or mentally—take a look back, reassess the terrain, and stop before you do damage to yourself or anyone else.

These stress-driven mistakes in performing routine tasks can run the gamut from locking your keys inside the car to forgetting to pick up the kids at school on your carpool day.

### What is Really Happening to You

> *I hated what I was doing, but I loved why I was doing it.*
>
> **—A daughter acting as her mother's caregiver**

Caring for a frail, dependent elderly person can cause emotional, psychological, and physical problems for you. No doubt about it: being a caregiver is tough. As your level of involvement increases, and your ailing relative's disease progresses, you will spend less time with your immediate family. Some of your friends will fall away, and you will cut yourself off from regular social activities.

As a primary caregiver, you face a much larger challenge if your loved one has dementia, which is present in 47% of those older than 85 years. As many as 80% of persons with dementia are cared for in their homes by family members. Caring for someone with dementia is associated with a higher level of stress than caring for someone with functional impairment from another type of chronic illness, according to a report published by the American Academy of Family Physicians (2000).

### Consider the Source

While you may feel that you are at your wit's end doing what is best for your elderly relative, consider that your loved one didn't choose to be in this predicament. Although some frail and ill individuals unconsciously added to their problems by not taking better care of their health when they were younger, most are declining through the natural aging process. To compound their physical losses with the possibilities of losing independence causes added stress to the care receiver, as well as the caregiver.

Estelle, who was introduced earlier in the chapter, thrives on the challenge of proving to her daughters that she must remain independent.

"I wish they'd all believe in me, and let me alone to see that I can live alone. Whether I fall or not … I still don't want to go to the hospital. They don't do anything for you there. If you don't have anything broken, forget it. You're home in a day or two. I have a doctor here that comes maybe four times a month because I have shingles. He really doesn't know anything about shingles. Nobody knows."

Although she guards her independence, Estelle also appreciates the time and attention that her family gives her. "Well, I value the time they give me, you know. They take time off to do something for me. Like my grand-daughter,—she does the shopping once in a while. She'll call and say 'hi'. I'll give her the list over the phone and then she brings it over or has it delivered."

*On the Road to Depression*

> *The next time my mother gets violent, I am calling 911!"*
>
> **—Deborah (pseudonym), adult daughter caring for her 82-year-old mother.**

An estimated 19 million American adults are living with major depression —the most common health problem for caregivers. Sixty-one percent of family caregivers providing at least 21 hours of care a week have suffered from depression, according to a study by the National Family Caregiving Association (1998). The illness is the result of intense sadness that interferes with the ability to function, feel pleasure, or maintain interest. Symptoms of depression include crying, interruption of sleep patterns, increased or decreased appetite, and lack of interest in family and social activities. Some studies have shown that caregiver stress inhibits healing.

### A Caregiver Seeks Help for Herself

*Rosemary (pseudonym) had a history of chronic depression. When her 80-year old mother moved into Rosemary's home, she knew she had to get help. "I saw my therapist right away." She was able to discuss her needs with her therapist and had an added blessing of getting her mother to talk with the therapist. "Mom resisted at first. Her mind was sharp and she was frustrated because she couldn't eat and couldn't walk. Her talking with the therapist helped."*

*As part of the sandwich generation—caring for an aging parent while taking care of her own children—Rosemary sought help for her 10-year-old daughter, too. "I saw attention being taken away from my daughter when my mother moved in. I instantly got her help. My daughter talked through her feelings with the therapist."*

Stress and the burden of care became apparent for Rosemary when her house suddenly felt crowded. "I was upset that I couldn't be alone in my own home. Sometimes you just want to be alone."

Losses are one factor that drives depression. For caregivers, losing control can include the loss of:

- Personal time
- Family time
- Privacy
- Social contacts
- Finances
- Energy because of the physical demands of caregiving
- Work outside the home
- Patience
- Self-esteem with feelings of failure as a caregiver
- Identity in shifting from a successful full-time worker to a daily in-home caregiver
- Self worth

The sense of loss is a two-way street. Care receivers, too, suffer from depression and can experience losses that they cannot easily control. The person requiring care is usually in this situation because of illness or physical limitations. While some losses to the dependent person are similar to those of the caregiver, some are very specific because of physical ailments. They may include:

- Independence
- Finances
- Privacy
- Social contacts
- Independence in self-care
- Outside-the-home activities
- Sense of life's meaning
- Sensory pleasure regarding smell and taste, sight, and hearing
- Mobility

Both caregivers and care receivers often feel put upon and forced into their roles. This loss of independence on both individuals fuels depression.

### The Long and Winding Road

In addition to resentment about giving up your own freedom and privacy to care for a loved one, there is a gray area that revolves around timing. In reality, you don't know when this caregiving job is going to end, or when—if ever—you will be able to get back to your life as it was. Knowing that you face a path of unknown length and uncertain destinations is an added cause of stress. Another source of stress is acknowledging that, whether you are doing a stellar caregiving job as the primary caregiver or one that is perfunctory, your parent is going to die on your watch.

### Role Reversal from a Different Perspective

Whether you are caring for an aging parent, extended family, or an elderly friend, you will probably experience an unsettling sense of role reversal. Essentially, your patient becomes the dependent child, and you become the manager and parent. You are now making the decisions, and you are giving advice to someone you love, who was independent, and whose advice *you* respected.

There are major differences between parenting your elderly family member and parenting a child. Your aging parent has a life history of experience and events to recall and a young child does not. Legally, your aging loved one has all his or her rights to decision making, unless you have established legal guardianship. There is a sense of hope in knowing that your child is becoming less dependent as time goes by, while you experience an added sense of fear as your parent becomes more dependent.

Family relationships are further challenged in this quasi role reversal context—especially if the care receiver and family caregiver are at odds from past family history. Often, both care receivers and care providers in this situation are filled with resentment, and in some cases, remorse. (An in-depth look at caregiver resentment is covered in Chapter 12.)

### Financial Stress

As if the emotional baggage of caring for a family member weren't enough, the financial responsibilities of caring for a frail loved one can add another layer to the stress factor. If you have your elderly parent move in with you, the financial responsibility of having another mouth to feed, more laundry to handle, and less time to yourself, adds to your stress. On top of all this, if you have to take time off from your full- time job, your financial woes increase exponentially.

According to studies regarding the economic impact of Alzheimer's disease on families, it was found that the average caregiver with a full-time job will miss more than three weeks of work a year, and that one fifth will quit their jobs altogether to provide full-time care.

### The Stress of Caring for an Aging Spouse

Spouses providing care for their husbands or wives make up 23% of the caregiving population. Caregiving for a partner in marriage is perceived as stressful by many because the caregivers themselves are often old and have health-related problems. If you are a caregiver over 80 years old, the cards are not stacked in your favor for you to continue living a healthy lifestyle. Elderly caregivers with a history of chronic illness who are experiencing caregiving-related stress have a 63% higher mortality rate than their non-caregiving peers.

### Male Caregivers versus Female Caregivers and Stress

In 2003, a Metlife survey of employees of Fortune 500 companies found that men were just as likely as women to say they cared for their parents. Males also experienced caregiver burnout. However, it was found that sons, as caregivers, reported significantly less of a sense of burden than did daughters or other relatives, according to research conducted by Faison, Faria, and Frank, (1999).

The reason behind fewer problems for males is, perhaps, because they are less involved in the more personal aspects of care, such as feeding, toileting, bathing and dressing. Instead, men, as family caregivers, are more likely than women to take care of the paperwork and financial matters of their parents.

### Caregiver Stress at Midlife

Your caregiving term is a period of transition—a time when you experience life changes due to the needs of, and responsibility for your ailing loved one. It is a life event that causes a role change and/or a crisis.

As we travel through life, there are a few inevitable passages. As everyone who lives to old age must deal with death and taxes, we must pass through the inevitability of middle life. For a vast number of individuals who encounter that middle-age juncture, the transition creates a period that is known as the midlife crisis. Ironically, the time frame for the majority of adult children who are caregivers falls during their midlife years. Author Nancy Schlossberg, Ed.D., defines a transition as "any event or non-event which results in changed relationships, assumptions and roles." It is also safe to say that, in the caregiving arena, an individual's relationships will change as well as his or her role.

In its simplest form, midlife crisis affects people between the ages of 40 and 60, and is often described as an individual's discontent with life, or with a lifestyle that may have provided happiness until this point. Symptoms run the gamut from questioning the meaning of life, ("Is this all there is?") to boredom, exhaustion, or daydreaming. Some people respond to midlife-crisis symptoms by acquiring a new and younger spouse, material objects, or services to hang onto the proverbial fountain of youth: a facelift, a shiny new Porsche, or maybe an extreme hair color to hide the gray.

Researchers are now finding that the task of caregiving can greatly increase the depression that individuals feel during their mid-life crisis stage. When midlifers have raised their children and expect the freedom that comes with becoming empty nesters, family care providers often find themselves with the added burden of caring for an aging parent.

Providing care during mid-life can be turned into a positive experience, according to Darby Morehardt, MSW, LCSW, and Director of Education at the Northwestern University Feinberg School of Medicine. "As a mid-life task, caregiving can provide the caregiver an opportunity for psychological growth, a chance to resolve earlier, unresolved issues with a loved one, and a way to face one's own mortality and renegotiate the adult child's relationship with the parent. It can be a time for healing and forgiveness."

### What Can You do About Stress?

Peggy, 66, a quadriplegic who received personal care from care providers for more than 41 years, had this advice about how care recipients can make their own family caregivers more comfortable. "Anything that you will do that will cut down on the feeling of being on instant call helps reduce the stress and then helps reduce the resentment, which makes the chore a lot easier for both of you. Some of the burnout that occurs in family caregivers has to do with not understanding what the other person is feeling. Hence, the caregiver often feels unappreciated. It's important to teach the aging parents to respect that."

*Get Counseling*

Fortunately, a wealth of information and resources for counseling options is available to caregivers. Some cost money, some are free. In the majority of cases, seeing a professional about caregiver stress will greatly reduce both the burden of care, and the feelings of guilt. An extensive list of agencies and resources about counseling for depression is featured at the end of this chapter.

Social workers and geriatric case managers can provide many resources and referrals to qualified specialists who counsel caregivers. In some cases the social workers themselves will provide counseling. The advantage of turning to social workers for help is, while they can provide referrals to counselors, they can also help assess and make suggestions about your individual caregiving situation. Your local hospital is an excellent resource for case managers, social workers and counselors near your home. Additional referral sources listed at the end of this chapter can direct you to help in your community. According to a study by Mittelman, Roth, Coon, and Haley (2004), of the New York University

School of Medicine, short-term intensive counseling, along with readily available support from counselors, had a positive impact on caregivers more than 3 years after the initial counseling sessions ended. In the study, published in *American Journal of Psychiatry*, when people taking care of spouses with Alzheimer's disease sought counseling, the caregivers' long-term risk of depression was greatly reduced. This positive effect on the caregivers continued even after a spouse with Alzheimer's died or was placed in a long-term-care facility.

### Find Humor Wherever You Can

I want to stress this point right up front. There will be situations when you will make ridiculous mistakes, and moments when your loved one's lack of cooperation will make you feel like crying. But if you can find the humor in those little nuggets of absurdity, perhaps you'll find yourself laughing instead. Even the most stressful situation can contain seeds of hilarity, sometimes even joy. Look for them, and savor each one.

### A Hysterical Moment

*One Friday night when my husband was working late, my parents and I went out for pizza at one of the local chain restaurants. We were seated in a booth, with Mom and Dad on one side and me on the other. The table in the booth was the kind that is attached to the wall, and sliding in and out can be tricky, with little room to maneuver.*

*My mom was at the mid-stage in her Alzheimer's journey, where she talked very little but laughed a lot. Our job was to cue Mom on a few of her daily tasks. She was able to walk and eat on her own, and always enjoyed an evening out. Mom was a large woman, carrying most of her weight in her midsection.*

*When it came time to pay the bill, my dad sped off to the cashier, as was his style. I slid out of my side of the booth and discovered to my horror that Mom was stuck. She had somehow wedged her belly between the table and the back of the booth, and couldn't budge. I coaxed her by taking her arm, trying in vain to get her to slide out.*

*It wasn't working. My dad was nowhere in sight. What made matters worse was that Mom and I started laughing hysterically. This made it even harder for her to concentrate and take the cue to slide toward freedom.*

*By this time, a waitress had arrived to help, and other diners were now offering their aid. There was a lot of commotion, which only confused my mom that much more. My dad came back to check on us. We declined the help of others and were able to bring some calm to the situation. Finally, we were able to coax her out of the booth. We laughed all the way home.*

The blessing? Mom was safe and unharmed, and she laughed through it all. By doing so, she calmed our fears. To this day, I savor my memory of this "nugget of joy."

### Turning Acts of Kindness into Real Action

When people say, "Take care," while it is surely meant with sincerity, they need a more dynamic way to express honest-to-goodness concern. It needs to be forceful, just short of a command. Friends who offer to help with "Take care," need to think of their offer as a directive, instead of an act of kindness. Your friends and family, who are generally concerned that you might drive over the edge, need to say, "Go right home and get some sleep." Or, "I'll be over at 10 A.M. tomorrow to stay with your mom, while you go and get your hair cut. Don't argue with me. Be ready to go by 9:45."

At a seminar I attended on grief counseling, the guest lecturer, whose brother had committed suicide, was adamant about accepting help from others during his time of grief. He called himself the "suicide survivor." He talked about one of his neighbors, who not only offered to grocery shop for the family during the days after his brother's death, but also went ahead and did it. She didn't wait for the family's permission and she didn't ask for a list. Every day, she brought over a quart of milk, sandwich meat, and all the essentials to keep the grieving family going. She *just did it.*

### Turning "How Can I Help" into Real Assistance

Be armed. Be ready. Give assignments. Whether you are in the epicenter of providing care or your loved one has just died, when someone asks how he or she can help, assign that person a job. It's okay to let go. It's okay to give up some tasks, and not continue to be "Super Caregiver." This is one baton that should be passed. Pull out your laundry list of things that others can do for you. I can't stress this enough. Most of your friends and family members who offer to help really mean it.

### Action Steps

*Go to the Source.*    It is a mistake to not include persons who need care in every decision. Their opinions matter. Their vote counts. Decisions about housing, care, and finances will be handled more easily if the care receivers are involved from the start.

When you are faced with an emergency situation where your charge has been rushed to the hospital, try to get someone else to drive *you*. Your emotions will be at their highest peak, and will hamper your own driving skills.

While you are writing down the emergency data, repeat the information to someone who is with you. Two sets of ears are always better than one when it comes to reacting after hearing bad news.

### When Depression Rears its Ugly Head

Notify your physician and be honest about your feelings and level of stress. Do a "brain dump" about everything that is going on with you. This is not the time to be shy or meek. If you don't have a physician or can't pay for one, check the public health center in your area. Look into a family service or social service agency. Many employee-assistance programs can make referrals to health care specialists. Most importantly, *don't face this alone*.

Consider respite care for your loved one. Many retirement communities, assisted-living facilities, and nursing homes offer respite programs. This is a short-term stay for your family member so you can get some rest and recharge your batteries. Look into a Caregiver Respite Exchange program through your local Area Agency on Aging. The agency's phone numbers are listed in local phone directories. You will be matched up with other caregivers in your area who have similar needs and need a break.

### Caregiver Help in General

Join a caregiver support group. Seek support from other caregivers. Know that you are not alone. When I facilitated a focus group of males who had been caregivers to a parent, none of the participants felt that they received any help from their families or friends. Most felt isolated in their role as caregiver. As one respondent wrote in his survey, "I thought I was the only one out there who had a mother who was ailing." You can find caregiver support groups through your local hospital, the Area Agency on Aging in your community, and through www.eldercarelocater.com. Call the Eldercare Locator toll-free at 800-677-1116. Monday through Friday 9:00 A.M. to 8:00 P.M. (ET)

Have a good laugh. Sometimes even the craziest circumstances result in a situation that is so funny we have tears rolling down our checks. The old adage that laughter is the best medicine couldn't be more on target. Laughter, like tears, is a form of release. It's a way to inhale a fresh breath of air. Take advantage of the moment. Laugh until your belly aches.

Avoid destructive behaviors. You know what they are, and know when you are most susceptible to bad habits. When you are stressed out over your caregiving roles, it becomes easy to overeat, have too much alcohol, medication, or cigarettes. These habits are all crutches. Face the stress head on, and don't let these bad behavior habits in the door.

It doesn't matter which organization you turn to for help. What is most important is that you take action and get yourself some assistance—as much or as little as you need.

### Where to Turn for Help

*The Family Leave Act (FMLA)*    The FMLA is a government-sponsored benefit allowing workers to take time off to recover from their own serious illnesses or to care for loved ones, including an elderly parent, without risking their jobs. Employees can take up to 12 weeks of unpaid leave per year through FMLA, which was signed into law on Feb. 5, 1993, by President Bill Clinton, and took effect 6 months later. More than 35 million workers have utilized the benefit.

Ask your employer or your human resources department manager about FMLA. Go to the Family and Medical Leave Act Advisor at www.dol.gov/elaws for frequently asked questions.

*Caregiver Resource Room*    The Caregiver Resource Room provides caregivers and professionals with information about The National Family Caregiver Support Program, including where you can turn for support, assistance, and services. http://www.aoa.gov/prof/aoaprog/caregiver/caregiver.asp.

*The American Geriatrics Society*    Articles about options for caregivers who care for family members with Alzheimer's disease. AmericanGeriatrics.org

*Resources for Dealing with Caregiver Burnout*    The Alzheimer's Association, 800-272-3900, or on the Internet at http://www.alz.org.
The Alzheimer's disease Education and Referral Center, 800-438-4380.
The Family Caregivers Alliance, 800-445-8106; http://www.caregiver.org
National Family Caregivers Association, 800-896-3650; http://www.nfcacares.org.
MEDLINE (www.ncbi.nlm.nih.gov) can be searched for information on Alzheimer's disease caregivers.
Powerful Tools for Caregivers classes, by MatherLifeways: Classes for family caregivers providing skills to improve self-confidence, reduce stress, communicate feelings, and cope with the love, guilt, loss, and responsibilities of caring for a sick loved one. 888-600-2560.

*Additional Resources*

Children of Aging Parents
800-227-7294/215-945-6900

National Association of Professional Geriatric Care Managers
1604 N. Country Club Road
Tucson, AZ 85716-3102
520-881-8008/520-325-7925 (Fax)
www.caremanager.org

ElderCare Online
Comprehensive library of articles, educational modules, and online support services for people caring for aging loved ones and the professionals who serve this community.
www.ec-online.net

National Association of Social Workers
750 First Street, NE, Suite 700
Washington, DC 20002-4241
www.socialworkers.org

National Depressive and Manic Depressive Association
730 Franklin Street, Suite 501,
Chicago, IL 60610
800-826-3632/312-642-0049/312-642-7243(FAX)

National Foundation for Depressive Illness
P.O. Box 2257,
New York, NY, 10116
800-248-4344/212-268-4260/212-268-4434(FAX)

National Institute of Mental Health
Public Inquiries, Room 7C-02
5600 Fishers Lane,
Rockville, MD 20857

National Mental Health Association
1021 Prince Street,
Alexandria, VA 22314-2971
1-800-969-NMHA(6642)/703-684-7722/703-684-5968(FAX)

Web MD
www.webmd.com

# CHAPTER 4

# Growing Old and Feeling Ill:
# A Permanent Condition?

## Stuck in a Body That Won't Cooperate

Has this happened at your house? The grandmother who used to be kind and smiling has become irrational, uncooperative, and somewhat ... annoying. It's not her fault. She is stuck in a body that is not cooperating. Your dad used to be this person who could multi-task, hold a full-time job, manage the family finances, and figure out the longitudinal equation for getting the space shuttle back into the Earth's atmosphere. Well ... maybe not that last one. Now he's telling his doctors how to do their job.

While these challenges may disrupt the harmony in your house, the bottom line is this: whether you are taking care of a friend or family member, you don't want them to suffer. In this chapter, the various diseases and ailments of the elderly are explored. We take a closer look at what can be done to ease the pain of care receivers and lower their level of anxiety. You will also find tips to lessen the impact of your patient's mood swings on the rest of your family.

We will look at fashioning the best possible relationship with the care receiver's physician. Better communication skills are suggested so that the ailing care receiver understands the diagnosis and feels that the medical appointment was a success.

The interaction between grandparents and grandchildren will be explored, as will as mood swings, changes in habits, and bad behavior.

*The city is too big and too bustling to accept older people, I think—unless those older people are very independent. And some*

*things you can be independent in, and some you show your depen-
dence. I walk with a cane, and the cane itself is an agent for both independence and dependence: For independence, because I can use it in a
threatening manner. It's dependent because I need it to walk with,
and it shows other community members that I need help. So it works
both ways. Well, I have no fear of letting people know that I need help.
I'm willing to help people and it's a normal expectation of mine that
somebody would give me help.*

—Jimmy, 85

*Slowing Down*

Many of the care receivers interviewed here acknowledged and accepted
that their own bodies were slowing down. Jimmy doesn't seem to mind the
slower pace. "It's a natural part of aging, I think. We still have a body, and
the body parts are weakening. Everything except an idea itself is a body
part. That doesn't mean that it quits, but it means the body is slowing
down and that takes some getting used to."

*The ailments of the elderly are, for some, their best topics for con-
versation. Estelle, 94, tells it like this: "People are nice. They say, hello,
how are you? Well, they don't ask anymore how you are. I can see that
it's bad when you ask me how I am. I say, 'I'm sick. I don't have to tell
you.' So, they don't say anymore, 'How are you?' That's bad. Who-
ever's going to listen to this is getting an earful.*

*Their Pain Is Real*

In the simplest of terms, the elderly experience more pain than younger
individuals because their bodies are wearing out. Chronic pain for the
elderly is real. By age 75 many persons exhibit some frailty and chronic illness. These individuals represent the oldest, sickest, and frailest portion of
the population. They also represent the fastest-growing segment.

Older people are more likely to suffer from back problems, arthritis,
bone disorders, diabetes, and a whole host of other diseases. A telephone
survey conducted by Louis Harris and Associates (1997) found that one in
five older Americans (18%) are taking analgesic medications several times
a week or more, and 63% of those had taken prescription pain medications for more than 6 months.

*I'm angry because I'm old now and I don't feel good and I can't do
anything because I'm sick. So, I don't know about old age. It's not any
good in a way, because you can't do the things that you did before. You
feel like you're cheated now. Because when (my husband) Henry died,*

*you know, I could have had more years with him. Then he got sick and died, so now he's dead over 10 years. If I wasn't sick, we would've had more time together. Oh, well.*

—Estelle, 94

Persistent pain brings on other negative consequences for our elderly including sleep disturbance, impaired ambulation, depression, anxiety, and decreased socialization. Individuals who experience pain when moving or walking are less likely to venture out to visit friends or attend social gatherings. Depression from isolation begins to set in.

### Depression Can be Fatal

The risk of chronic pain's leading to depression is very real. What is more disturbing is that severe depression can prompt individuals to take their own lives. People over age 65 have the highest suicide rate of any age group. It is estimated that 20% of elderly (over 65 years) persons who commit suicide visited a physician within 24 hours of their act, 41% visited within a week of their suicide and 75% have been seen by a physician within 1 month of their suicide.

Risk factors for suicide among older persons differ from those among the young. In addition to a higher prevalence of depression, older persons are more socially isolated (U.S. Dept. Health and Human Services).

*I did not understand any of this, and I did not want to understand. The diagnosis was horrifying. First I thought it was an almost instant death, which I could prepare for. Then I found out I could live many, many years, like Ronald Reagan. That was beyond horrifying to me. I did not want to be an automaton. I wanted to die, and quickly. I was strongly suicidal, but I tried to cover it from my family. I went down very deep into a pit that I felt was built by me. Nothing was right.*

—Les, diagnosed with Alzheimer's disease in 2000

### More Involvement and Knowledge Means Less Pain

Keeping care recipients involved and informed about every step of their pain management is critical. Studies show that when patients are exposed to education programs combined with self-management and coping strategies, their overall pain management is significantly improved. There is evidence, too, that older adults with good coping skills experience lower pain levels.

Gather all the brochures and articles you can find about your charge's specific pain problems. Discuss interventions and other options such as experimental drug studies, support groups focusing on specific diseases, or moving from traditional health care practices to holistic practices.

### My Dad and Self-Diagnosis

During my father's elderly years, he became actively involved with his own diagnosis and his physician's recommendations, because my dad read everything he could get his hands on about his particular ailments. My father had also studied Latin in his earlier years, so with a medical dictionary and his limited knowledge of Latin, he felt he had the upper hand regarding prescriptions. Sometimes, much to the physician's chagrin, my dad went a little over the top trying to be part of the medical team. However, that was all right with me and my siblings. He was interested, involved, and he concentrated less on his pain.

## Geriatric Medical Care—Not a Top Priority

A vast number of medical professionals maintain opinions and attitudes that limit their ability to perceive the needs of the elderly.

- Ageism—the term for discrimination against older people—is still very much alive in the U.S. health care system. Older patients are routinely overtreated, undertreated, or even mistreated by health care professionals with little or no training in geriatrics. Some physicians believe that elderly patients, because of their age, can't tolerate surgeries or radical treatment that could stop the spread of some diseases. Other medical professionals feel that surgery on a patient at this late stage in life is just a waste of time.
- In this day and age, many physicians seem to believe the older patients cannot understand diagnoses or recommendations for care, and, during a medical appointment, still focus their discussion and attention on the elderly person's family member or caregiver instead of on the person involved.

These approaches can be validated and proven true or false only on a case-by-case basis.

Les, who was introduced earlier, believes that the doctors he now sees for his Alzheimer's disease treat him as an equal team member. "Finally, I think we are making a mark on the doctors who treat us. Most importantly, I am now always included in the discussion with my wife, Barbara, the doctor, and me. If there is one thing [to remember], the patient should not be marginalized, Alzheimer's disease or not."

*Making the Visit to the Physician a Success*

If the care receiver doesn't have a primary care physician or a geriatrician (see below), ask for references from other elderly friends and relatives who are happy with their care. Hospitals all have physician referral banks.

Opening up the lines of communication between the elderly care receiver and the physician and asking the right questions is critical. Bring all the current medications along to the office visit. Encourage patients to tell the physician about everything that is bothering them—even if it seems trivial. The physician needs to get the whole picture.

A program funded by Pfizer Inc., called Partnership for Clear Health Communication, suggests several strategies to help patients to get clear directions from their health care providers. The organization suggests that these three questions are critical for a patient to ask his or her physician:

1. Why is my pain a problem?
2. What do I need to do?
3. Why is it important for me to do this?

A brochure from The Partnership for Clear Health Communication suggests:

> "If you, or your elderly loved one still don't understand the diagnosis or treatment, you need to take responsibility and continue to ask questions. Don't be embarrassed or feel rushed if you don't understand something. You have the freedom to ask your doctor, nurse, or pharmacist as many times as you need to."

Here are a few tips that will further open up the lines of communication between elderly patients and their medical professionals:

1. Ask the three questions listed above.
2. Have a friend or family member accompany the elder to the doctor's visit.
3. Together with your care receiver make a list of health concerns to discuss with the doctor or nurse.
4. Bring a list of all current medicines to the doctor or nurse.
5. Ask a pharmacist for help when there are questions about medicines. The advantage of asking pharmacists is that one is available by phone 24 hours a day.

*In Praise of Geriatricians*

Just as you would turn to a medical specialist for advice about heart disease or cancer, the same should be true in the field of aging. That expert is a geriatrician—a physician who looks at all of the individual's symptoms, medical conditions, medications, and preferences. While a cardiologist focuses on heart disease and an oncologist treats cancer, the geriatrician creates a care plan to treat all of the symptoms that present themselves for the whole of the aging patient. He or she is a specialist who considers the patient's age, physical history, psychological history, and environment. A geriatrician is trained to handle the multiple interacting conditions, drugs, social situations, and psychological problems that an older person may face.

Is it always necessary to call in a geriatrician for an aging person? In a *Boston Globe* (2003) article, Dr. Lewis A. Lipsitz, vice-president of academic medicine and co-director of the Research and Training Institute at Hebrew Rehabilitation Center for Aged in Boston wrote, "Not every older person needs a geriatrician; however, every physician needs some training in geriatrics. Unfortunately, few physicians have the skills or resources necessary to properly address the medical challenges presented by many elderly patients."

Currently there is great need for more physicians who make geriatrics their specialty. Compared with the large resource pool of physicians in other medical fields, the numbers of geriatricians are significantly lower. Geriatricians represent 1% of all physicians, or approximately 9,000 specialists who are expected to treat the 35 million persons 65 and older (one for every 3,888 older persons), according to the Alliance for Aging Research (2002).

> *I have been independent for so many years, but now I've become dependent for people to take me to the Jewel for groceries, or to Walgreen's for medication, to the bank. I feel bad, because I did it on my own. I wish I could do that. Come next summer, I hope I can do it. Yes, I hope so. I pray so hard that I'll be able to walk to the Jewel.*

**—Ann, 92, was sidelined from her independent lifestyle when she took a bad fall. Her favorite physical activity is walking. She hopes to be out enjoying her walks again very soon.**

## Thinking Positive

Elderly patients who described themselves as highly optimistic had lower risks of all-cause death, and lower rates of cardiovascular death than those with high levels of pessimism, according to an article in *Archives of General Psychiatry* (2004).

Over a period of 9.1 years (1991 to 2001), participants who were ages 65 to 85 years (999 men and women) were tested to see whether individuals who are optimistic live longer than patients who are pessimistic. Compared with participants who reported a high level of pessimism, participants reporting high levels of optimism had a 55% lower risk of death from all causes, and a 23% lower risk of cardiovascular death.

"We found that the trait of optimism was an important long-term determinant of all-cause and cardiovascular mortality in elderly subjects independent of socio-demographic characteristics and cardiovascular risk factors. A predisposition toward optimism seemed to provide a survival benefit in elderly subjects with relatively short life expectancies otherwise," according to Erik J. Giltay, M.D., Ph.D., of Psychiatric Center GGZ Delfland, Delft, The Netherlands.

> *Oh, it makes me feel bad that I have to ask for help, you know. 'Cause I figure they're giving up their time to wait on me or do something for me. So, I'd rather not ask them to do anything. That goes for friends and family and everybody.*

—Estelle, 94

*When Grandchildren Feel Their Pain*

If you have young children or teenagers, it is important that they be included in the circle of care for the ailing care receiver. Whether your aging parent lives with you, or you are caring for a neighbor down the street, your children need to understand what part they will play in the care. They also need to know the signs and symptoms of the particular disease and have a general understanding of your caregiving time commitment.

When it is the child's grandparent who is ailing, having the grandchildren involved will often bring comfort and hope to that person. Getting visits from children usually helps an elderly person forget pain for a short period of time and reinforces the bond between the child and the grandparent.

Young children should be told openly and honestly about the symptoms their loved one is experiencing, including tremors, lack of coordination, or forgetfulness. Incontinence and unpleasant odors should be discussed honestly, and should be explained as part of the aging process.

Children can also do their part in making a safe environment by not leaving toys, books, or shoes in an area where the care receiver could trip and fall. Perhaps there are certain times of the day when visits are more appropriate for children, when the patient isn't taking medication or feeling tired.

It is critical for children to understand that their grandparent's symptoms are part of the disease and not a reflection of a changing personality. They also need to know that the symptoms do not indicate that the grandparent no longer loves the child; the love and understanding in the relationship are still very much intact.

Acknowledging that your elderly loved one is in pain will help them feel that they are not alone. In turn, helping your children through this journey as their grandparent suffers through an illness will ease additional stress within your household. Every elderly individual deserves the best medical services and personal care available to ease suffering.

- Look for ways to help steer parents toward a positive attitude. Perhaps they can become interested in journaling about their past lives, or become reflective on changes in lifestyle they have experienced over the years. Get them to talk about the best years of their lives.
- When looking for medical expertise for your elderly loved one, seek out geriatricians who specialize in the care of the elderly.
- Bring your spouse and children into the circle of care. Explain to family members that any anger or unusual behavior by ailing parents may be a symptom of their disease.
- Be honest with children about the symptoms and side effects that their grandparent may be experiencing during this illness.

CHAPTER **5**

# Getting Up Close and Personal

*My caregiver needs to be honest, strong (I need someone who can lift me), caring, self-motivated, and computer savvy. One who can learn to understand my distorted speech. And finally, one who can give a urinary catheter or be able to learn how.*

— George, 76, suffering from the
advanced stages of Lou Gehrig's disease

## Things No One Wants to Talk About

Bodily functions, loss of control, adaptable equipment, incontinence, eye matter, organ malfunction: they're not always pleasant conversation topics, but they are very much a part of everyday life for a wide range of older individuals, especially those with declining health. Does your elderly relative have constant halitosis because of disease, a sinus infection, medications, or difficulty with oral hygiene? Or, does he just have bad breath because he has lost his sense of smell, and continues to overload his meals with onions and garlic? Topics in this chapter are personal, private, and not for the faint of heart.

Few people discuss the nuisances and inconveniences that produce poor hygiene because a body part is malfunctioning. This chapter tells readers what to expect when dealing with personal care. Even proper foot care regarding toenails, eye matter, and body odor are part of everyday maintenance to keep a body fine-tuned.

Family caregivers still provide 80% to 90% of all personal and medical-related care to elderly relatives. Armed with the proper knowledge, caregivers can address the personal care issues of their loved ones. There is a certain cadence that can be created in the delivery of care if the care receiver and the caregiver are working in tandem. The end result? The tasks are accomplished more easily, and the care receiver feels fit as a fiddle—or at least ready to receive visitors.

If an elderly parent is transitioning through his or her final days, the proper hands-on care administered by a loved one can bring a sense of peace and comfort to the dying relative. Hospice workers, who are already trained in personal-care skills, are a wonderful resource to tap into during your relative's last stage of life.

> *I need a full-time caregiver to get me out of bed, transfer me from my chair to and from the vanity, the shower, my auto, the john, and on occasion, to clean my behind. He has to dress and undress me, help with meals, act as translator, give me a catheter when I cannot urinate … I could go on and on.*

> —George, 76

## Before the Personal Care Begins

Two important concerns need to be addressed before any hands-on or supervisory personal care happens: issues of maintaining the recipient's dignity, and knowing how to administer every task in the correct way. For your elderly relative's emotional and physical well being, each of these issues need to be clearly understood before any assistance takes place, and then monitored and reevaluated as care progresses.

The next few pages explain the limits some receivers face in managing their bodily functions. Care receivers as well as caregivers are introduced to various support groups that deal with ostomies and bladder and bowel malfunction. Communication strategies, dignity issues, and resources for emergency and long-term help are discussed.

### Dignity

Talk to your ailing relative up front about personal-care issues. If he or she is uncomfortable about having you or another family member assist with personal tasks, explore resources from home health agencies. Paid caregivers can give people who are modest about their privacy a sense of independence. They also relieve them from the worry of "not wanting to be seen like this" by immediate family.

If cost prevents your family from bringing in paid help, check into resources through various charitable agencies or your own Area Agency on Aging. Many provide services on a sliding scale, according to income level.

*Discussing the Problem*

Individuals who experience personal health problems such as incontinence, sexual dysfunction, or personal-hygiene difficulties because of an illness often are very reluctant to discuss their problems. They are embarrassed or humiliated because they don't have control. Trying to hide their embarrassment about incontinence or poor hygiene only makes the situation worse.

During their formative years, the World War II generation did not openly discuss intimate personal matters. It is only because of the barrage of media messages and advertising-brand blasts that words such as "acid reflux," "constipation," "feminine hygiene," "gingivitis," "hemorrhoids," and "sexual side effects," have been added to our everyday vocabularies.

You can help your elderly patient feel less isolated by the problem if you speak in general terms about how many people have similar problems. Figures on the percentages of older people who suffer from the same problem is good information to share. Referring to role models or celebrities on television who have similar problems and have gone public with their symptoms may help your care receiver open up.

When actress June Lockhart of the popular 1950s television show "Lassie" appeared in a television commercial for an incontinence product, she piqued the interest of a new and different audience. Famous jazz musician B.B. King has appeared in TV ads admitting that he has diabetes as he pitches a particular glucose monitor, and Senator Bob Dole has even introduced the subject of erectile dysfunction through his television ads touting Viagra.

Many older individuals from varied walks of life have ostomies due to intestinal and colonic problems. The late Queen Mother of England; Marvin Bush, brother of President George W. Bush; Al Geiberger, pro golfer on the seniors tour; and Rolf Benirschke, former place kicker for the San Diego Chargers, have all had ostomies.

*Bathing*

While the majority of the able-bodied population takes regular bathing for granted, for someone who is physically challenged or suffers from dementia, taking a bath can be a major ordeal. Issues about modesty, privacy, and dependency make the experience uncomfortable for someone who has recently become dependent.

When the individual has dementia, they are apt to feel less trust for the caregiver because the bathing task is foreign to them. According to Levine, Reinhard, Friss Feinberg, Albert, and Hart (2004), the caregiver may encounter disruptive behavior, particularly when the care recipient feels confused, threatened, or insulted, or if he or she is physically uncomfortable. The care recipient may perceive certain acts, like being moved into the bathroom, undressed, and washed, as physical or sexual abuse and may respond with combative behavior. If the care recipient suffers from arthritis or other mobility problems, he or she may resist going into the bathroom because movement is painful.

> *I found another way to get into the bathtub. I don't sit in there. Because I did that one day and I couldn't get out. I couldn't get out of the bathtub. I take a bath and I kneel, on my knees, and then I wash my hair. I'm flexible enough to do that.*

> —Ann, 91

Even when the care recipient is more passive, bathing can present difficult challenges. Because the body deteriorates and loses its resiliency and elasticity with age, an older person's bones are more prone to fractures and breaks.

> *I accept help with no problem. It is no strain whatsoever on me. For instance, they help me bathe now. Well, I don't want to fall down in the tub. She helps me get into the tub and cleaned up. And one of [the aides] said recently that I was the only one they had seen in a long time who was perfectly relaxed with it—that most people stiffen up, or reject it, or don't need a bath, or something like that. Well, I realize that I do need help. And it has to come from somewhere, and I would rather it come from someone who has some training.*

> —Jimmy, 85

The best way to help dependent persons with personal-care issues and to be able to intelligently discuss their concerns is to be armed with information. Listed below are definitions of several of the physical conditions mentioned in this chapter.

*Terms You Should Know*

**Halitosis:** The unpleasant odor carried on the breath. It is usually the result of gum disorder, tooth decay, smoking, or indulgence in aromatic foods. For the elderly, halitosis can be brought on through aging, certain medications, diseases such as diabetes, dental problems, and physical difficulty with oral hygiene.

**Incontinence:** Loss of bladder or bowel control. It results from a lack of control in the nervous system, commonly occurs in the young, the elderly, and those with illness or mental impairment. Incontinence may be caused by a disorder of the urinary tract (including infection, bladder stones, or tumors) or by prolapse (displacement) of the uterus or vagina in women.

**Ostomy:** The surgically created opening in the body for the discharge of body wastes. A stoma is the actual end of the ureter or small or large bowel that can be seen protruding through the abdominal wall. The two types of ostomies that are referred to most often are colostomy and ileostomy.

**Colostomy:** The surgically created opening of the colon (large intestine) that results in a stoma. A colostomy is created when a portion of the colon or the rectum is removed and the remaining colon is brought to the abdominal wall.

**Ileostomy:** The surgically created opening in the small intestine, usually at the end of the ileum. The intestine is brought through the abdominal wall to form a stoma. Ileostomies may be temporary or permanent, and may involve removal of all or part of the entire colon.

**Sexual Dysfunction:** In older men, erectile dysfunction (ED) usually has a physical cause, such as disease, injury, or side effects of drugs. Any disorder that causes injury to the nerves or impairs blood flow in the penis has the potential to cause ED. Between 15% and 25% of 65-year-old men experience ED. Some men experience this condition due to prostate cancer treatment. Women experience changes as they grow older, with urinary-tract infections occurring more frequently. Women also experience a thinning of the vaginal wall and reduced moistness in their sexual organs due to a decrease in estrogen.

**Urinary Catheter:** A urinary catheter is any tube system placed in the body to drain and collect urine from the bladder. Urinary catheters are sometimes recommended as way to manage urinary incontinence and urinary retention in both men and women. Catheter care by caregivers should first be taught and supervised by experienced health care professionals.

## Halitosis

Although halitosis can occur because of gum disease or tooth decay, among the elderly in long-term-care facilities, extreme bad breath may be caused by lack of regular dental hygiene. For those residents who need assistance with teeth brushing, their daily hygiene rituals may be compromised if the nursing homes are short staffed.

If you are in a situation where your care recipient is at home, make an extra effort to pay attention to oral-hygiene needs. Too often, because of poor eyesight and limited hand and arm range of motion, the brushing of an individual's teeth isn't accomplished on a consistent basis. Sometimes a cupful of mouthwash used alternately with the tooth brushing can solve some of the bad-breath problems.

## Eyes Wide Open

Cataracts, glaucoma, and age-related macular degeneration are the three most common eye diseases that lead to blurred vision in the elderly. Another problem that isn't half as critical as the previous three, but should get some attention, is eye matter. Because elderly individuals don't retain as much moisture in their bodies as they grow older, small dust particles and mucus tend to collect and dry out in the corner of each eye. The easiest way to maintain good eye hygiene is to gently wipe away the eye matter with a damp, clean washcloth.

## Incontinence

Toileting and accidents involving incontinence are some of the most sensitive conditions that an elderly person can face. As mentioned earlier, your elderly relative may deny that there is a bladder-control problem, or hide it because it is difficult to admit loss of control of this area of life. Incontinent elderly individuals also don't want to be reminded to change their incontinence products because it draws attention to their problem.

> When I have to go to the washroom, I can't hold it. My kidneys are weak. They don't come quick enough. They are overworked. They won't let me stand alone, so I can't get to the bathroom myself.
>
> —**Charlotte Z. 94, who relies on nursing-home staff to take her to the bathroom**

In some instances, modern technology and its incontinence products works against solving the problem. As one adult daughter told me, "My mother won't change her Depends™ when they need to be changed, because she doesn't believe they are wet." The daughter said that, because of their advanced technology, Depends incontinence pads have a stay-dry lining that keeps the wetness away from the wearer's body. As a result, this elderly care receiver believes that she doesn't need to change the pad with any kind of frequency, and it becomes overly saturated.

## Ostomy

Having an ostomy and wearing a device to collect waste from the colon is not a problem for all ostomites. Whether your elderly relative has a colostomy or an ileostomy, acceptance and living a quality lifestyle depends on attitude, according to David Rudzin, treasurer of the United Ostomy Association, head-quartered in Irvine, California. "In most cases, when you have to go in for the ostomy, you are really sick, and when you come out, you are just happy to be alive. It's all a mindset. I would advise anyone who has an ostomy to be patient. In many cases, you feel like you are the only one who has one."

### Support Groups

Individuals who are in situations with personal-health conditions that create a burden in their lives often feel isolated. Finding help through like-minded individuals in the same situation often brings a new perspective to the problem.

Rudzin said about ostomy support group, "If an individual is not comfortable with his situation, he should find a support group of other folks with ostomies where people understand you. People can live really normal lives and play sports, swim, and have intimacy. It's all about atti-tude. This is what you have; it's not who you are."

When George, 76, was looking for help about his avoidant paruresis con-dition, he found a support group, but was unable to attend because his ALS symptoms made him homebound. Also known as psychogenic urinary retention, avoidant paruresis is a social anxiety disorder that involves the inability to pass urine in the presence of others. It can start at any age and affects mainly boys or men, although girls and women can also suffer from it.

Although he couldn't physically get out, George however, did not become discouraged, but utilized his next best resource, his computer, to access the support group. "If only I had found the avoidant paruresis web site, an international paruresis organization (Bashful Bladder Phobia) ear-lier, and had been able to desensitize myself and not be bothered with this nuisance. There are desensitizing support groups in major cities now, including Chicago. But I'm not physically able to attend their meetings. I do go to their chat lines."

Relying on a positive attitude about one's own health care can also keep fears about various treatments at bay. Despite his rigorous schedule, Clif-ford, 77, who has diabetes, doesn't complain. He leaves his assisted-living apartment three times a week to receive dialysis treatments. Each treatment takes 3 hours. "There's nothing to be afraid of with the treatment. The hard-est part is sticking yourself with the needle (to monitor his insulin levels.)"

### Proper Foot Care

Brittle toenails are common in elderly people because of their tendency for poor circulation. Deformed or brittle nails should be trimmed and examined by a podiatrist. Having an elderly person maintain his or her own toenails could present a problem and a safety issue. If the individual is already in declining health with poor eyesight and difficulty bending due to stiffness or arthritis, he could do serious physical damage by trying to trim the toenails on his own.

> *The nursing home where Charlotte lives doesn't have a podiatry office, or special chair for residents' foot care. "They come and they get me down on the floor and cut my toenails. I get a manicure every Friday, too. If I want my nails clipped, I have to get special permission. The guy comes in and I have to sit on the floor. They help me down, and they get me up."*

—Charlotte Z., 94

### Hiding Infirmities

For the elderly to fiercely guard and maintain their independence, they will often conceal their infirmities from others. In retirement and assisted-living communities, residents tend to do more socializing in common living rooms and game rooms than in their own apartments, mainly to socialize with other people. A second, subliminal, reason to stick to the common areas is that the individual's apartment would reveal more about their needs and gradual loss of independence: a raised toilet seat, crumbs and spills that can't be seen due to poor eyesight, a commode next to the bed. If the dependencies are even more severe, such as incontinence that can't be managed, the elderly person will begin to withdraw from social events.

### The Conflict of Care

When differences regarding care occur between an elderly relative and a family caregiver, health care professionals try to listen to the concerns of both, and choose the best intervention to move forward with care. In turn, by lacking common sense, caregivers and care receivers are often at odds about the best possible care when their decisions are driven by pride, emotion, or cost.

For Glenn Ulffers, DDS, it was no surprise that the majority of his dental patients were elderly, considering that for 17 years his Chicago dental office was attached to a skilled nursing facility. Dr. Ulffers witnessed first-hand the conflict between the desires of the adult child and the wishes of his or her elderly parent regarding dental care. "While the adult child wanted all of the latest procedures performed on his or her parent to ensure healthy teeth, the elderly parent resisted. The elder would say to me, 'Just do what is necessary for now. I am old, I am not going to live that much longer.' For each of my patients, I respected their wishes and only performed the procedures that they wanted."

At times, an elderly parent's physical condition has changed as a result of something psychological or emotional that is happening in their lives. In these instances, the interventions to cure the physical conditions often don't solve the problem. This example has occurred with some of Dr. Ulffers' patients. "The elderly parent would stop eating, and in many cases, was losing his or her desire to eat. The children saw this as a sign that the parent needed new dentures. There were many reasons why new dentures were not the 'cure-all.' For some, the elderly parent didn't want to wear dentures at all. In most cases, however, the parent had just lost the desire to eat."

> *There comes a time when you have to know how to accept the responsibility of your position. And try to live it. You just don't want to be constantly reminded of the fact that, 'I had to put your diapers on you. Now, I've got to sit here while you put your diapers on me.' It's a very hard two-way street, but it's something that has to be done. It sometimes will be quite upsetting, but you're the parent now. Don't be afraid to accept responsibility.*

—Jimmy, 89

*Action Steps:*

Make your relative's dignity one of your first priorities. Always follow the lead of your ailing relative. Respect privacy and confidentiality.

- Any type of personal health care needs to be done the right way. If you are assisting your ailing relative with hands-on personal care, ask plenty of questions before you help out. Call your family member's doctor's office and find out all you can about your tasks.
- Wear latex gloves. In the event that you are going to come in contact with waste, body fluids, or blood, always wear appropriate gloves. You will lessen your risk of picking up an infection.
- Help your family member research support groups and websites for information about specific problems. As mentioned earlier in the chapter, support groups for urinary incontinence and ostomies are valuable resources for individuals with those specific conditions.

If there ever was a time to imagine yourself walking in someone else's shoes, it is when you see loved ones in their most vulnerable state. Take a look at their kaleidoscope of care. Try to see their resistance from a different perspective. If it is confusing to you, think about how daunting it is to the person whose health is being chipped away a little bit each day. Allowing loved ones to still be "whole" people will help them maintain their dignity. They need to be in charge of their independence. No matter what their current health dictates, they need to feel physically and emotionally complete.

# CHAPTER 6

# Driving Through the Fog

*How frightening is it to drive through a dense fog on an unknown dark and winding road, having no clear picture of what dangers lie around the bend? That is Alzheimer's disease.*

### Navigating the Clouded World of Alzheimer's Disease and Dementia with Grace and Happiness

Since being diagnosed with early stage Alzheimer's disease, Jenny Knauss has experienced her own artistic "renaissance." Her passion for art, combined with deliberate mental concentration, has fueled her talent for pencil sketching. She frequently sketches flowers and sculpture at the Art Institute of Chicago. When patrons of the art museum stop to admire her work in progress and ask her how she is able to produce such marvelous sketches, she is tempted to reply, "First, you have to have Alzheimer's."

Jenny is 68. A native of Melbourn, U.K., she graduated from Somerville College at Oxford University. She worked on her Ph.D. thesis on West African history in the period before that area's independence from British rule. She was a lecturer in the History Departments at both the University of Ibadan, Nigeria and the University of Ghana. She has spent more than 30 years in health advocacy.

As a result of her diagnosis in April 2002, Jenny is now passionately advocating for earlier diagnosis of Alzheimer's disease, as well as support programs and services to meet the needs of persons with early stage dementia. She is a member of the Early Stage Support Group Program for Persons with Alzheimer's at the Cognitive Neurology and Alzheimer's Disease Center at the Northwestern University Feinberg School of Medicine in Chicago (CNADC). Together with her husband, Don, a Ph.D., physicist and patent agent," Jenny has taken her message about early detection to many advocacy forums, including the Alzheimer's Association Policy forum in Washington, D.C.

She and Don have created Alzheimer's Spoken Here, Inc., a not-for-profit corporation. Both their company and website, www.alzsh.net, were created with the mission to give persons with early stage Alzheimer's disease a voice, and to produce educational materials created by persons with Alzheimer's.

While Jenny spends much of her time on advocacy work, some of her day-to-day functions have fallen away as a result of the disease. With the help of Don, as her primary caregiver, Jenny skillfully works around those tasks she can no longer handle. She is unable to operate a cell phone or a computer. She doesn't operate household gadgets. Her cooking is limited to heating water in the microwave oven for tea, and the only housekeeping chore she tackles is vacuuming the floors. Don works very hard to create a stress-free home environment for Jenny.

One deliberate change Jenny made in her life to create less stress—and subsequent agitation resulting from her disease—was to leave her job as executive director of the Illinois Caucus for Adolescent Health. She had become forgetful on the job and increasingly agitated over her mistakes.

Although Jenny Knauss has very few fears about her future as the disease progresses, she voiced concern about her personal care: "I certainly would hate to be cared for by someone who didn't understand me," she said. "Or by someone who thinks that, because I have Alzheimer's, my head has gone completely awry. If people would come in and fuss around, it would be annoying."

In reference to the assumptions many people make about the disease, Jenny added, "I find it obnoxious to make assumptions about someone else's life."

### What is Alzheimer's Disease?

Alzheimer's disease, like cancer and AIDS, is among the cruelest diseases known to humanity. It is an irreversible, progressive brain disease that slowly destroys memory and thinking skills. As it progresses, Alzheimer's disease generally takes away an individual's ability to perform such daily activities as bathing, dressing, walking, and toileting. Some sufferers lose their ability to swallow. While Alzheimer's disease spares its victims the actual physical pain that cancer patients endure, the mental and emotional suffering it inflicts on them and their family members is devastating.

*Dementia* is an umbrella term that describes the symptoms of a person's changes in thinking, memory, language abilities, and visual/spatial abilities. It can also mean a change in personality or behavior. Alzheimer's disease is one of the most common forms of dementia. Other forms are vascular dementia, frontal temporal dementia, and Lewy body dementia.

At present, about 4 million people in the United States have been diagnosed with Alzheimer's disease or some other form of dementia. It is estimated that 14 million Americans will have Alzheimer's disease by 2050, unless a cure or means of prevention is found. Most individuals diagnosed with the disease are over 65 years old. As people grow older, they have a greater risk of getting the disease. Almost half of people over age 85 have Alzheimer's or related dementias.

*What to Look For*

Ten Warning Signs of Alzheimer's Disease:*

1. Recent memory loss that affects job skills
2. Difficulty performing familiar tasks
3. Problems with finding the right words
4. Disorientation of time and place
5. Poor or decreased judgment
6. Problems with abstract thinking
7. Misplacing things
8. Changes in mood or behavior
9. Changes in personality
10. Loss of initiative

As is the case with Jenny, it isn't unusual for people who have been diagnosed with early Alzheimer's disease to know exactly what is happening to them. Some individuals choose to continue their normal lifestyle without making adjustments. Many actively participate in their own fight against memory loss, work outside the home, and even continue to drive. Those who choose to fight the disease are relentless in finding as many resources as possible about the disease. Many individuals drastically adjust their diets and commit to a healthy lifestyle. Some make adjustments within their own environments to eliminate as many stressful situations as possible.

## Going Public

My mother knew she had Alzheimer's disease long before her official diagnosis at age 75, and she knew what to expect. She had witnessed her own

---

* Source: Alzheimer's Association

mother's regression as she traveled through the various stages of the disease for 10 years. My mom willingly gave up driving at her doctor's request, and wasn't timid about sharing her diagnosis. When neighbors and friends from church would stop her in the grocery store and ask why she hadn't been to various meetings and social gatherings, she responded, "I have Alzheimer's disease."

President Ronald Reagan found it critical to go public with his diagnosis. "At the moment I feel just fine. I intend to live the remainder of the years God gives me on this Earth doing the things I have always done."

Convincing the former First Lady of Australia, Hazel Hawke, to announce publicly that she was diagnosed with Alzheimer's disease required a bit of prodding from her daughter, Sue Pieters-Hawke. In *Hazel's Journey: A Personal Experience of Alzheimer's*, Pieters-Hawke writes,

> *"Although Mum is naturally reticent about personal difficulties, and also worried that people might see her as a 'silly old thing, losing her marbles', she was drawn to the idea of going public if it would decrease the stigma of the disease and help others. She just wasn't convinced it really would do any good. It's that terminal modesty again!*
>
> *"She listened to us, thought about it and finally said, 'I think you're probably overrating the difference I could make, but if you really think it could be useful then yes, bugger it, I'll do it.'"*

Hazel Hawk made her announcement in November, 2003. "Although I would obviously prefer not to have Alzheimer's, I continue to live a happy and healthy life, with love and support of family and friends. I hope that, by speaking out about this very private issue, I can help to promote openness, awareness and support for all people living with dementia. No illness should carry a negative label. None of us is immune."

For Mary Lynn "Sydnee" Conway, a flight attendant for American Airlines who retired after 39 years of service, her church pulpit became her platform for announcing her diagnosis. "Very early on I decided that if I had Alzheimer's, I'm just going to tell everybody. I went into church one day and I took the mic[rophone] and I said, 'Now don't fall down, and don't faint, but I have Alzheimer's!' And everyone was looking at me like, 'AH!' Well, that's the best way around it. Just get it out. Now when I walk into church, everybody comes up and kisses me.

*"The more friends you have around ... and that means there are more people around you who will speak out and ask, 'Are you tired today?'"*

*The Need to Know*

Informing people with early stage Alzheimer's about their diagnosis represents a shift in thinking by the professional medical community. According to Darby Morhardt, director of education, Northwestern Alzheimer's Disease Center: "The notion that individuals couldn't really understand their diagnosis or disease has been challenged over the last several years. So there's this big movement to tell people their diagnosis, if they are asking … and even if they are not asking. There is more and more recognition that people do have an awareness and an understanding of what's happening to them and want to talk about it. They can benefit from that support from other people. You have to tell someone they have the illness before they can make some shifts in their lives that they wouldn't have otherwise made."

For some individuals, a diagnosis of early stage Alzheimer's serves as a "wake-up call" to begin to live life differently. Morehardt said some people try reinventing themselves and experience a newfound freedom. For a select few, the onset of the disease is seen as an opportunity. According to Morhardt, four typical reactions and actions follow early diagnosis:

1. Some individuals slip into a depression.
2. Some believe an opportunity has presented itself.
3. A few make a conscious decision that life with the disease is not so bad.
4. Some believe they don't really have the disease and go into denial and depression.

Les Dennis, 68, is a mover and shaker who received his Ph.D. in Global Human Resources at age 61 from Chicago's Loyola University. Over his lifetime he has traveled to every continent. When he was diagnosed with early stage Alzheimer's disease in January 2000, he was so devastated by the news that he became suicidal. To add to his grief, his 15-year-old granddaughter, Wendy, died of cystic fibrosis that same year. Les was diagnosed just 2 years after he retired from Loyola. "I was horrified and pretty down. I was ready to go into the water."

The water Les refers to is Lake Michigan in Chicago, a few blocks from where he and Barbara, his wife of 47 years, currently live. Their home, just south of downtown, is complete with Les's bountiful garden. Prior to his diagnosis, Les had many occupations: paper boy, freight handler, railroad clerk, labor leader, CIA operative, graduate- and high-school teacher, lobbyist, and finally professor at Loyola.

The worst time of Les's journey was in the early days of the disease. "I didn't know what Alzheimer's was. I was suicidal and took antidepressants. I overdid it."

Les sought help from a support group in the suburb where the couple lived at the time. "This place was full of crazy people," he says. "All of the members of that group were in denial. They discussed a lot of kid stuff and said things like, 'I can't do this, I can't do that.' I wanted to do other things. I got the hell out of there."

He found a whole different environment in a new support group he joined, Chicago's Northwestern Cognitive Neurology Alzheimer's Disease Center (CNADC), where Jenny Krauss is also a member. Like Jenny, Les had spent the majority of his adult life doing advocacy and civil rights work. It is perhaps not surprising that he soon became one of the best advocates for early detection. "Our support group at Northwestern is really a wonderful thing," he declares. "It surprised me at first. We help each other out and we are a comforting group. Our group meets in one room and the caregivers meet in another. We are people with Alzheimer's. We have crazy parts to it, and we laugh a lot."

When Les first joined the CNADC support group, those diagnosed with the disease and their caregivers were meeting together in the same room. Les quickly became dissatisfied with this arrangement and demanded a change. He told the coordinator of the group that he would quit if they combined the two groups again. "We had to stand and wait until the caregivers were done talking," he says, "and we had to sit next to the caregivers and all that bull—. They say things like, 'We shouldn't do this and that.' Now the group has really become our own."

At this point in our discussion, Les pulled out a large meat cleaver that he used during a panel discussion to dramatically emphasize that he still has the ability to prepare food for cooking. "The caregivers think we can't do much of anything," he says. "We still have the capabilities and can do lots of things. "We're a happy group. The caregivers can't figure it out. We are so happy with each other. You don't have to explain everything to each person in the group. There is a different dynamic."

*Knowledge is Power*

"This may sound ridiculous, but I feel like I've been empowered now, more than I was before," says Sydnee. At 61, she has been living with the knowledge of her disease for 2 years. "I've learned so much along the way. I feel like I can do it better than somebody else."

Sydnee's positive, take-charge attitude keeps her smiling in the face of adversity, and her spirited generosity lights up the room. If a friend or former co-worker were to be diagnosed with Alzheimer's, she would be a pillar of support. "I would say, 'Come on over. We'll take out some tea, and … no crying. I just want to know how you're going to handle this. And I'll be right there behind you. I've been through all this already, so you can just sit with me.'"

She would offer encouraging advice, too, to any adult child whose parent had been diagnosed with Alzheimer's. "First, I would suggest that he get another medical opinion. An adult child can reach a parent by making the parent be as comfortable as they can be." Even if the subject matter is difficult to talk about, Sydnee believes that the more knowledge a person has, the better off he or she is. "There's lots of information. I would ask if they know anyone else who has the disease so that they could speak together."

Sydnee first realized something was wrong when she became very forgetful both at work and at home. "One minute I thought I put something in the oven, turned around, and thought, 'Did I put that in the oven'? At work things were getting out of hand. I finally knew, 'This isn't me.'"

As you talk with Sydnee, you see only glimpses of her symptoms. As you engage her in conversation, she will suddenly stop talking, and then resume with a polite, "Where were we?" or, "What were we talking about?" These brief moments are only incidental. They do not define Sydnee as a human being. Her courage, her compassion, her positive outlook—these are the things you remember.

### After the Diagnosis—Choosing to Change Your Life

For Jenny Knaus, getting the diagnosis was a welcome relief because she knew something was wrong, but she couldn't get a handle on it. "I became interested in it. Understanding (the diagnosis) gave me something tangible. It helped keep the 'beast at bay'. I became interested in issues around the disease."

As with Jenny, many individuals who are diagnosed and living in the early stages make positive adjustments in their lives. Morehardt told of one woman in her CNADC support group who immediately implemented lifestyle changes when she was diagnosed. 'This now helps me make some plans in my life that I wouldn't have otherwise made,' the member said. Morehardt added, "This particular patient and her husband have gone ahead and are traveling and spending time with their family. They are not working."

One positive element that Les believes the disease has brought into his life is a sense of caring more for others. "All that comes from the (CNADC) support group," Les says. "I realized I could do other things and help others." He adds, "I was always helpful. Working very hard. Now it's different. I am trying hard to learn that things are okay." Les continues to be forthright in taking charge of events, but is also practicing patience in letting life unfold.

Some individuals with Alzheimer's bump up their travel plans to take full advantage of the lucidity that remains in the disease's early stages. Since Len's diagnosis, he and Barbara have traveled to Antarctica, the Mayan ruins, Portugal, and Belize. On a desk in his den and home office is a travel tome punctuated with dozens of Post-It® notes marking the places they have traveled to and those they plan to visit. The book is appropriately titled, *1,000 Places to Visit Before You Die* (Schultz, 2003).

Sydnee and her husband, Lino Darchun, plan to travel for as long as they are able. "Actually, I am really blessed with Lino, because he loves to cruise," she says. "We love to take trips. The more things you see in this world, the more fun you have."

### Is it Forgetfulness or Alzheimer's Disease?

If you have a history of Alzheimer's disease in your family, each time you forget a family member's name or miss an appointment, you fear that the disease has set in. The difference between forgetfulness and Alzheimer's disease is simple. Forgetting an appointment or misplacing an object is a temporary loss. Not knowing what the purpose of the object, or having any recognition about the date, could be a symptom signaling the onset of Alzheimer's disease. For example, not being able to remember where you left your gym shoes is forgetfulness. Not knowing what the gym shoes are for, or which part of the body the shoes fit, could be Alzheimer's disease.

### Fears and Frustrations

Fear of the unknown is what paralyzes us into depression and despair. To lose lifelong memories is frightening beyond words. For my mother, who had the disease for 7 years until her death in 1999, Alzheimer's was *not* an unknown path. She had seen her own mother suffer with the disease for 10 years. This glimpse of her own future both alleviated and exacerbated her fears. She anticipated that she would have many of the same symptoms that her mother had experienced—speech aphasia, memory loss, and incontinence. Her most unsettling fears, like those of many other Alzheimer's sufferers, were of the uncertainty about the duration of the disease and the severity of its symptoms.

One of Mom's fears during the early stages was not knowing whether her words were going to come out in coherent sentences. Her early symptoms included the progressive misuse of words. This was an especially worrisome thought for a woman who was not only an ace accountant, but also an avid reader, a champion Scrabble player, and a crossword aficionado who completed puzzles every day.

She voiced her fears to my sister and to me prior to the celebration of her 50th wedding anniversary. She hadn't been sleeping at night because she was worried about her interaction at the party. "What if people come up to me, and I don't know what to say?" she would fret. We suggested that she acknowledge her guests by telling them that she was happy that they were there. We also reassured her that we would stay by her side for the entire celebration.

My mother's symptoms were not unique. First, she lost her ability to organize words. Her verbal skills regressed and she eventually stopped talking altogether. She became incontinent. For the last year of her life she was bed bound and unable to communicate. She lost her fight with Alzheimer's disease and died of pneumonia in 1999.

Losing the power to make decisions is a primary fear for Les Dennis as his Alzheimer's disease progresses. "I want to make sure that I can do what *I* want to do. I also want to quit when I know I should."

*Frustrations with the Medical Community*

Both Les and Jenny are frustrated about how patients with Alzheimer's disease are handled by medical professionals. Jenny's primary concern is for those people who go undiagnosed and those who don't have access to quality screenings, medications, and specialists in the field. "Early diagnosis is rare, unless you have access to good specialists and programs like those at Northwestern," she says. "I worry about people with Alzheimer's disease who are in less fortunate areas like [Chicago's] north Englewood. "People who speak limited English don't understand the issues around early diagnosis. It should be routine rather than rare."

Concerning physicians in general practice, Jenny becomes adamant about their knowledge regarding early diagnosis. "Physicians don't understand it. Physicians are ancient. Alzheimer's has not always been considered a health issue. It swings between a mental and physical issue. The physicians are not looking for problems with the brain. We need to get to the elderly docs who haven't caught up."

Les minces no words when it comes to offering advice to physicians who treat Alzheimer's patients. "First of all, if you are a medical type, shut up and try to listen to the patient. You might actually learn something of value. If you are a patient, be assertive. You must make them realize that you are a real live person. If you do not get answers, find a better doctor." As Les's primary caregiver, his wife Barbara advises other caregivers to verbally remind doctors to speak to the patient, not the caregiver. "Too often, the caregiver is talked to, and the patient ignored. You have to position yourself right next to your spouse in the examining room so that the doctor can address you both at the same time."

One symptom of the disease that frustrates Les is his inability to be comfortable in large groups. Les and Barbara, who have two sons and five grandchildren, have made adjustments in their family life to deal with his concern. "What we are doing differently is not having the grandchildren and children here all at once," he explains. "It got chaotic for me. Now we see them in smaller groups."

Friends of Les and Barbara deal with Les's diagnosis in different ways. "Friends fall off when they find out," says Les. "People with Alzheimer's are slow. The loyal ones stay. Many of my students still come over. We go out."

## For Patients, Caregivers, and Others Dealing with Alzheimer's and Related Diseases

Says Les: "Having kicked you around into the reality of this disease, let me now give you some ideas I have picked up from others with AD."

*Les's Ideas for Coping*
- *Get out of the house. Walk. It will help you mentally and physically.*
- *Stay away from big groups; noise and bewilderment can throw you down.*
- *If you are confused, befuddled or lost, people will help you. Don't be afraid, but use discretion.*
- *Your friends are your friends. Tell them what's happening to you.*
- *Many (oh so many!) acquaintances will pull the drill of "we all for-get things now and then." Remember, this is AD. Their experience simply is not the same as our disease.*
- *Get into a support group.*
- *Doctors are people, and many know little more than the average person does about AD.*
- *Travel!*
- *Life, of course, does end. For me, the idea of somehow transfiguring myself into a sort of walking nice guy with no discernible cogency is not my cup of tea. I have decided that life for me will end when they try to use life support systems. Complete advanced directives or durable powers of attorney for health care.*
- *The other side of life can be beautiful for quite a while. Remember, most people with AD are having longer life spans.*
- *The first part [of the disease's progression], however, is the best. Don't waste it with denial or pretending. Go for it. Meet with your kids and tell them about what is happening. Enjoy them. See more of them.*

—Leslie E. Dennis, Ph.D.

*Looking at The Future*

As his disease progresses, Les knows that his ability to live an active life will be cut short. The time will come when he is no longer able to make decisions or function physically or mentally on this own, and for this he has established his end-of-life plan and is confident that his family will honor his wishes. "I have a system all prepared. My sons and Barbara know this is what I want. Basically, if I can't talk, I don't want to live, and they all understand. It was a hard time. It still is hard for Barb."

In an article he wrote for *Perspectives—A Newsletter for Individuals with Alzheimer's or a Related Disorder*, Les reflected on changes he has made with respect to family members and communication about the disease, "I have changed through all of this. I walk a lot. I have had discussions with my adult children about marginalization, reminding them that us old folks still want to be part of the party. Preteens and teenagers, of course, know everything, but that has always been their domain."

Syndee is not worried about what lies ahead. "We're really in a very wonderful position the way the technology is now. For medications, taking care, and for getting your stuff up to par." She adds that she doesn't dwell on the future. "I don't worry about it too much now. But I know this is the kind of disease that doesn't go where I want it to go." Lino is Sydnee's support person and primary caregiver. "Lino's really good about making sure that … he goes and checks my pills. I turn around and say, 'You already did that', but, I figure if I don't take those pills, it's going to be a problem. I'm pretty good about taking care of them."

> *I told my younger sister, if you've got the [Alzheimer's] gene, you can't fix it. It's not going away. I'm comfortable and enjoying my time of life. In the future, a caregiver may have to be hired, to be around. Help me out. Walk the dogs when I am not able. I may need a caregiver to see that I'm ok. I didn't want it. But I'm not kidding. What do you do about it? Just have a good time."*

> —Sydnee Conway

*What to Do When It's You*

You've been diagnosed with Alzheimer's disease. Now what? Keep your brain fit … it's not too late. Look into research on nutrition, hormones, and medications. Read everything you can about moods, attitudes, and outlook, and how they affect your memory.

- Keep your environment safe. Look toward your future and decide how you will get help when needed.
- Reassess your work situation, and consider your short- and long-term options.
- Investigate some of the new drugs on the market. ARICEPT® (donepezil hydrochloride) is used for early stage Alzheimer's disease. Namenda has been shown to be an effective treatment for the symptoms of moderate to severe Alzheimer's disease. It is believed to work by attaching to the NMDA receptors in the brain and regulating the activity of glutamate, helping to ensure that the right amount of glutamate is available. Glutamate helps create the chemical environment needed for the brain to process, store, and retrieve information, resulting in learning and memory.
- Get your affairs in order regarding Advance Directives, including health care, power of attorney, living will, and organ donor information.
- Get into a support group. Look for a similar group for your family members.
- *Good health, good health, good health.* Get plenty of exercise, stop smoking, and don't consume excessive amounts of alcohol.
- Watch your diet. Go low-fat, and include the recommended amounts of vitamin E and folic acid.

Proponents of Vitamin E consumption believe that symptoms of Alzheimer's disease and dementia may be offset by taking 1,000 IU (international units), twice daily of the vitamin. A New England Journal of Medicine (1997, April) study suggested that the deterioration of patients who have moderately severe Alzheimer's might be slowed through treatment with vitamin E, selegiline (Eldepryl), or both. Similar studies that appeared in the Journal of the American Medical Association (JAMA) suggested that vitamin E obtained from food may be associated with reduced risk of Alzheimer's (2002). The antioxidants vitamin C and beta-carotene, according to this study, did not reduce the risk.

Scientists may have reversed their stance on the effectiveness of vitamin E however, because of new studies from the Johns Hopkins School of Medicine and the Bloomberg School of Public Health, (Nov.2004). Researchers found that people taking high doses of vitamin E (in excess of 400 IU) may in some cases be more likely to die earlier.

*Brain Food*

Numerous studies suggest that a healthy diet, including the following foods, will keep the brain healthy and slow the progression of Alzheimer's disease:

**Colorful fruits and vegetables.** Five servings a day. Spinach, kale, broccoli, blueberries, strawberries, and oranges. Benefit: All contain antioxidants that fight damage to brain cells.

- **Fish.** Two to three servings a week of oily fish. Salmon, halibut, mackerel, trout, and tuna. Benefit: Fish is rich in omega-3 fatty acids.
- **Nuts.** Almonds, walnuts, and pecans. Benefit: Nuts contain antioxidants that may fight Alzheimer's.
- **Foods to avoid.** Any food high in saturated fat, such as butter, processed foods, fast food and anything fried."

Don Moyer credits the healthy diet that he and Jenny Krauss adhere to, as much as the medication Jenny takes, for slowing down the progressive symptoms of the disease. Their diet regimen includes no meat, daily high quantities of fish with omega-3, and lots of antioxidant vegetables.

*Consider This*   Research released in November, 2003 clearly shows that those who consume food or supplements rich in omega-3 fatty acids have a 40% to 50% reduced risk of developing Alzheimer's disease. There is also clinical evidence that antioxidants, which are free-radical fighters, are effective in preventing and beating back the symptoms of both dementia and Alzheimer's, according to a report that appeared in *JAMA*. On the basis of the study, practitioners added high-dose vitamin E supplements (2000 IU daily) to their standard treatment regimen for Alzheimer's. The study further provided evidence supporting the concept that vitamin E, as well as vitamin C, has a role in delaying the onset of Alzheimer's disease (*New England Journal of Medicine*, July, 2004)."'

*Delaying the Onset—Keeping Your Mind Sharp*

Mental stimulation has been known to slow cognitive decline and to help reduce the risk of dementia in old age, according to numerous studies. I am referring to mental exercises to keep your mind sharp. Brainpower increases as your activities increase. Various ways to increase brain power, sometimes called *brain aerobics*, include challenging the brain to

---

" Source: Alzheimer's Association
"' A study by John Hopkins University researchers, referenced earlier in this chapter, suggests that patients taking high doses of Vitamin E may, in some cases, die earlier than individuals not taking vitamin E.

new topics: word games, social interaction, taking classes, and travel. Individuals should try activities that will allow the mind to wonder and release creativity.

When Les Dennis first experienced the loss of his computer skills as his disease progressed, he took on the challenge of retraining himself to regain his computer keyboard technique. Les worked tirelessly to type one sentence per day onto the computer screen. Through his aggressive persistence, he was able to recapture his ability enough to craft his autobiography.

For Sydnee, keeping her brain as stimulated and as active as possible means being a voracious reader and worker of crossword puzzles. "I started them once I realized that if I wanted this head to work, I'd better start using it," she says. She laughs as she talks about the irony of Alzheimer's, and how she is astonished by people's lack of knowledge about current events. "I will go out with some of my friends for lunch and say something like, 'I can't believe what's going on in Fallujah,' and my friend will say, 'What's Fallujah?' I say, 'What the hell ... where've you been?'"

"I read all the time," she adds. "That keeps me going and that's what keeps my brain going."

As a result of the disease, Syndee no longer uses the computer. She does very little cooking. She has also lost interest in oil painting. Still, Sydnee's daily moments of joy come from immersing herself in activities that she loves—her gardening, and romps with the overly affectionate Becca and Katie, her Tibetan and Wheaten Terrier pups. Sydnee prefers spending time each week volunteering by serving meals to the community's homeless at the Dignity Diner, a program offered by her church. Becca and Katie accompany Sydnee and Lino to the diner and to church each Sunday. During the holiday season, you will find Sydnee wrapping gifts for the Barnes & Noble Bookstore charity drive.

These special moments of selflessness bring Sydnee considerable satisfaction and help keep her mind as sharp as possible, rather than bemoaning what she can no longer do. "I'm not playing Pollyanna," she says. "There isn't anything I can do about it. I may as well enjoy myself for as long as I can." It's this attitude—this immense personal courage—that has helped her face these difficult years with grace and, yes, happiness.

### If Not Alzheimer's Disease, What Else Could it Be?

Research has now been done on individuals who exhibit symptoms of Alzheimer's disease—such as poor balance, memory loss, and incontinence—and who have subsequently been misdiagnosed. Dr. Harold Rekate, a neurosurgeon at the Barrow Neurological Institute in Phoenix, has made great strides in recognizing a condition called normal pressure hydrocephalus, or NPH, which is caused by excess fluid on the brain. The pressure caused by this fluid triggers Alzheimer-like symptoms. The problems that occur for an individual with NPH fall into the area of gait (or walking), thinking clearly, and bladder control. According to Dr. Rekate, a surprising number of cases go undiagnosed and untreated.

Medical professionals now estimate that between 5% to 10% of the 7 million people in the United States who have been diagnosed with Alzheimer's disease may actually have NPH.

*Is it Alzheimer's or NPH? How to Find Out*    To get the best and most accurate diagnosis, a patent must get an MRI scan, which could cost between $2,000 and $3,000. The results of the MRI must be analyzed by a neurosurgeon who is familiar with NPH.

If the condition is NPH, it can be treated with a 45-minute procedure in which neurosurgeons surgically insert a tube, or shunt, into the brain. The tube drains the excess fluid from the brain and moves it to the stomach, where it can be absorbed. Patients who have had this procedure quickly regain their ability to perform their regular daily activities.

## The Next Phases

The individuals who spoke out about Alzheimer's disease in this chapter were all in the early stages and thus able to articulate their concerns and opinions. As the disease progresses, such people lose more mental cognition and symptoms that are more debilitating, including pneumonia and upper respiratory infections, pressure sores, fractures, wounds, and nutritional disorders, will occur.

In anticipation of the final phase of the disease, individuals should have their affairs in order and make their wishes known regarding extraordinary methods for extending life (such as gastrostomy, intravenous hydration, and the administration of antibiotics). The lines of communication should also be open with the individual's surrogate decision-makers, physicians, and family with respect to advance directives.

## The Lucky Ones

The individuals who contributed to, and who are referenced in this chapter—Mary Lynn "Sydnee" Conway; Leslie E. Dennis, Ph.D.; Hazel Hawke; Jenny Knauss; my mother, Dorothy McClenahan; and President Reagan—were all fortunate to be diagnosed in the early stages. They were able to take an active role in decisions about their care and treatment. All shared a willingness to be proactive about the disease. As Jenny Knauss so aptly put it, "Finding out (about having Alzheimer's disease) was a step forward. You can deal with what you know. You can't deal with what you don't know."

Jenny believes that your best advocate against the disease is you. "Get on with your life, and find out as much as you can about Alzheimer's disease—and FIGHT! Tell your friends. Talk about the disease. If you get a diagnosis, your life doesn't close down. Push to make sure that people like us are getting the most attention."

Through her advocacy for early detection, Jenny found a new mission. "It gave me the beginning of a new career. I was lucky. I was invited to speak at the National Alzheimer Convention in Washington, D.C." She concluded by telling me that she has more meaningful work still to come. "Alzheimer's does not take up all of my life."

# CHAPTER 7

# "Give Me the Keys"

## How to Say Those Four Tough Little Words to the Parent You Love

My dad's car. Not only was it his ticket to ride, it was his vehicle to personal freedom. He could go wherever he wanted to go. To most males born in the Depression era, their cars represented their legs. *My wheels,* as they called them. Many of these men started driving before the legal age of 16. Women born during that time were not exempt from this newfound method of independence. One of our interviewees received her driver's license by mail at age 13, and never took a driving test until she was 80 years old.

> *"How many people do you want to kill?"* That's the tough question Les Dennis poses to members of his early Alzheimer's group who insist on continuing to drive. As an individual who suffers from Alzheimer's disease himself, Les has become an advocate who encourages his fellow group members to give up the keys. *"Most people are outraged [when you tell them they should not drive anymore]. They say, 'I can still drive.'"* After a stern dose of persuasion, most comply with giving up the keys. *"They've all mellowed, and recognized that they can't drive anymore."*
>
> Les knew it was time to stop driving when, one by one, his adult sons requested that he not drive with his grandchildren in the car. *"I realized pretty well that something was wrong. I would be too far in front, or too close in back. We had just bought a new SUV to take our little granddaughters around."* The coaxing from his family for Les to stop driving hurt his feelings in the beginning. *"We don't have a car now. We have taxi vouchers that we use."*

A car is not only a near necessity for most of us, it has become an icon of rugged American individualism. For many elderly people, dwelling in a personal universe that's growing ever smaller, it's the last gasp of self-sufficiency. *I drive, therefore I am,* they may as well think. And as loving children of these parents, we sympathize. Sometimes we sympathize so much that we're loath to take away this final treasured vestige of independence.

Sadly, though, failing to take away the keys from Mom or Dad could be the biggest mistake we ever make. It could actually cost a life. Here are examples of three horrific incidents that underscore the need for timely intervention. These headlines shout out the grim realities of the tragedies that can occur when an elderly, impaired driver is behind the wheel:

*July 17, 2003: Death Toll 10 in L.A. Crash, Elderly Driver Probed LOS ANGELES (Reuters)—One day after an 86-year-old man lost control of his car and barrelled for three blocks through a crowded street market in Santa Monica, the number of dead rose to ten on Thursday as police considered possible charges against the driver. Eight people, including a three-year-old girl, died at the scene of the accident and dozens of people were hurt, many of them critically.*

*Two people have since died at local hospitals, an official said. At least two of those critically hurt were children, among them a 7-month-old boy who suffered major head injuries and other trauma.*

*Dec. 27, 2001: A 76-year-old man was driving a van that abruptly accelerated into a busy intersection in Manhattan's Herald Square, killing seven people and injuring at least eight.*

*March 29, 2001: A 73-year-old man who suffered a fatal aneurysm drove off a busy road in South Park, Pennsylvania, and into a walking path, killing three people. A passenger, the man's wife, was also killed.*

There are enough stories like these and statistics about accidents involving older drivers to fill volumes. Here are just a few statistics that drive home the point. They paint an arresting picture of older drivers.

- Drivers ages 65 and older have higher crash-death rates per mile driven than all groups except teen drivers (IIHS 2003).
- Motor vehicle-related deaths and injuries among older adults are rising. During 1990–1997, the number of deaths rose 14% and the number of nonfatal injuries climbed 19% (Stevens 1999).

- During 2002, most traffic fatalities involving older drivers occurred during the daytime (81%) and on weekdays (72%); 75% of the crashes involved another vehicle (NHTSA 2003).
- Rates for motor vehicle-related injury are twice as high for older men than for older women (Stevens 1999).
- Age-related decreases in vision, hearing, cognitive functions, and physical impairments may affect some older adults' driving ability (Janke 1994).
- The 65 and older age group is the fastest-growing segment of the population; more than 40 million older adults will be licensed drivers by 2020 (Dellinger 2002).

### Why is Your Aging Relative Becoming a Risk on the Road?

Does any of this sound familiar to you? Have you noticed that your mom has run into the curb a few too many times?

The poor driving habits that develop in elderly persons are directly related to the physical changes that happen as they enter old age. As people transition through the last third of their lives, their vision, reaction time, physical strength, hearing, and, in some cases, mental acuity, greatly diminish. According to research from the American Association of Retired People (Straight, A. and McLarty Jackson, A., 1999), reaction time decreases by almost 40% on average from age 35 to 65. Changes such as these make older individuals' driving ability less sharp and less accurate than in their younger years.

> *"I guess they thought it was time. I didn't think so (at the time) and I still don't. My license is still good until April. I have never had a ticket. Never had any problems. It was horrible. This is the only dependent thing that is irking me at this point. I cannot go where I used to go. I cannot do what I used to do. I either have to take a bus, or take a cab, or depend on other people. It's very irritating." She had been driving, without having an accident or a moving violation, for 74 years.*
>
> *Charlotte's family encouraged her to give up driving when she was seriously ill during the summer of her 91st year. "Everybody was on my back." As she tells it, she stopped driving to keep harmony in the family. "I said to them, 'If I live, and I am well, I will give the car up.' I made that promise, and I kept it ... not that I wanted to because I could still drive up until this point. I was so anxious to get well that I was willing to do anything. I've had a very unusual life. I can't settle down now."*
>
> **—Charlotte, 91, still fiercely independent**

*More Facts to Consider*

Physical strength and flexibility need to be at peak level when driving in order to turn and look through "blind spots" when backing up. Additionally, checking mirrors and being able to look around the car in a 180-degree radius is critical. This type of physical movement can be hampered with the onset of arthritis and stiff joints.

- Vision and hearing are two critical senses that need to be at their peak for the ultimate safe driving experience. One should be able to see both close up and at a distance, and must also have sound night vision and peripheral vision. One common vision problem for older adults is macular degeneration, which affects an individual's central vision and ability to see detail.
- Hearing is equally important, in that a driver needs to be sharply aware of train signal bells, horns, and sirens on the road. Loss of hearing is one of the most common conditions affecting older adults. One in three people older than 60, and half of those older than 85, have hearing loss.

*When It's a Matter of Life and Death: How To Take Away the Keys and Put on the Brakes*

*Time to Hit the Tough Love Button with an aging parent*    A car should be considered a lethal weapon. It is a loaded gun fueled by at least 15 gallons of highly flammable liquid. Sit down on a kitchen chair. Think of 1-gallon containers, 15 of them, all containing gasoline, lined up in front of you on your kitchen table. Think of yourself climbing up on top of the containers while someone pushes the table around the kitchen. It's a scary proposition.

Here's another arresting fact. If you are driving a car at 50 mph and you hit another car head-on that is also traveling at 50 mph, it is the equivalent of driving your car into a brick wall at a speed of 100 miles per hour.

When my dad was teaching me to drive 35 years ago, he also drilled into my head this little fact about exactly how much tire surface the car has to work with to come to a screeching halt. He held out his hands, palms up, and explained that any 2000-pound car only has four surfaces the size of four hand palms to make the car stop. That's not much rubber to stop a moving vehicle at 50 mph, or at any speed, on pavement. Do the "crash test dummies" know about this?

*Thinking in Reality Mode*

Let's reverse your elder care situation, and put another scene in front of you regarding who is beyond the wheel. Suppose, for a moment, that your

16-year-old son is exhibiting the following physical deficiencies and characteristics of conduct. This week he:

- Has had trouble with his vision and slow reflexes.
- Drove the car when he was specifically told not to for medical reasons
- Had a lapse in judgment for any number of debilitating reasons, i.e., alcohol, tiredness, drugs, (prescription or illegal).
- Believes he is a better driver than you know him to be.

If any of these symptoms or courses of conduct were present with your teenage son, you would ground him, take away the keys, take away the car, and sit on him if you had to. If there is any immediate danger, you must stop an elderly person from driving.

*More "Reality" Mode*    The same tough love needs to be applied to an impaired elderly parent. Your aging person has to be scooped up and tethered into the safety net of reality for his or her own sake, for the safety of others, and the sake of your sanity. The best possible scenario is to have an honest discussion where you both agree that ceasing to drive is the best outcome.

*The Non-Negotiability of Tough Love*    In the majority of cases, the decision to have an elderly parent stop driving is not negotiable. By the time you have to insist that he or she get off the road, there is no margin for saying, "You can drive if you stay within a mile of the house." Or, "Only drive between 10 a.m. and noon." Unsafe driving is an issue of black and white, or life and death.

**How Do You Take Away the Keys?** *When there is an Immediate Need* You have to take immediate action if any of the following have occurred:

- A physician has given the order.
- There has been a serious crash.
- Your loved one has been diagnosed with dementia that has progressed to the point where his or her decision-making capabilities have become impaired.
- Reaction time has been severely altered.
- Vision is severely impaired.
- He or she is taking medication that causes drowsiness or nervousness.
- He or she has a diagnosis such as uncontrolled diabetes or epilepsy that could cause loss of control.

*What if the Need is Immediate and You Meet Resistance?* The following tips may seem pretty drastic and cruel, but you are dealing with life and death.

- Show the person arresting headlines in the media describing accidents that have involved elderly, impaired drivers.
- Report your loved one to the authorities. He will have his license taken away.
- Disable the car. There are ways to have the distributor cap disappear, or ignition wires to become disconnected. Consult your local mechanic or a friend who knows what he is looking at under the hood.
- Make the car *go away.* Donate it to one of several charities that now welcome the donation of a used car. Usually the donation can be included as part of a tax write-off. Remove it from the accessibility of your loved one. Don't make this a hide-and-seek game. Do not notify authorities or the insurance company that the car is missing. Cancel the insurance policy when the time is right.

*One Who Gave 'Em Up*

"I was just afraid of being one of the ones where people would say, 'That's the guy that shouldn't be on the road!' You look on the street and there are so many people who are in trouble. I don't want to be one of those people who are talked about." Don, 77, hasn't driven a car for 7 years. He suffers from diabetes and is confined to a wheel chair, having lost his right leg just above the knee to the disease in 1997. He decided, during his recovery, that he would no longer drive. He said the decision to stop was solely his own. "I didn't trust (my ability) enough. I had to stop."

Don had been driving since he was 15 years old. "It was sad. No longer could you just go and see places. It doesn't stop you right away, because you've been in the hospital (after the amputation) and you are just happy to be out." Don admits that he is a bit of a procrastinator. Although he stopped driving immediately after his leg was amputated, he didn't sell his car until 3 years later.

Don is single, is a retired assistant high school principal and teacher, and holds a Master's degree from the University of Chicago. He has always led an active life, belonging to many organizations including Kiwanis, and loves attending the opera, concerts and many community events. He lives with his brother, Jack, 85, who is also a bachelor. Don added, "It wasn't bad. It was easy to go out. I thought, 'My brother has the car. He doesn't have children.'"

Shortly after his leg was amputated, Don was fitted with a prosthesis, and tried to get used to it, but there was too much discomfort and difficulty with blisters. "I felt sad, because it cost a lot of money." He also considered learning to drive a car equipped with hand controls, but chose not to move ahead with that type of arrangement. "Other people have those scooters. That's something I have thought about."

"As we both get older, I am getting the feeling that I would like to drive again because I'd like to go out on my own. Most of my friends are older now, too. It's difficult. For example, right now, Jack drives me, but he also has to fold the wheel chair and lift it into the trunk, and he's 7 years older than when this first started. My friends who have driven me in the past have gotten older, and they shy away from having to deal with the wheelchair."

To offset the strain of having to lift and stow the wheelchair each time they venture out, Don's brother recently bought a handicap-accessible van that has an automatic lift. Don is able to wheel himself onto the lift, and transfer himself into the van using the remote control. While the amenities of the van are many, an able-bodied person still needs to fasten the wheelchair securely into the locked position, using a number of safety belts.

Don acknowledges the difficulty of having his transportation needs fit into other people's schedules. "For example, I imagine, men and women who are in couples. You usually do things together. We are different, and we like to do different things. I go to church every Sunday, and am picked up by a woman who picks up a number of people. Jack and I go to different churches, so this works out well. I am hoping to find a younger person who can help me and drive me."

What Don misses most about no longer being behind the wheel is the spontaneity to get up and go. "Places you want to go to see that are beautiful. I hear of something wonderful to go to, and you have to ask someone to take you."

Don lives in a suburb 30 miles south of Chicago. He has access to public transportation that is handicap accessible. It costs $2.25 roundtrip. Its schedule is limited to weekdays until 3:30 p.m., with no service on weekends. Although Don has used this service in the past, he needs to have assistance arranged at home to get through the doorway of the house. The drivers of the transportation service are not allowed to assist people into their homes.

*The Not-So-Immediate Need*   A single occurrence of bad judgment, such as a missed turn, a lack of proper signaling or getting lost, does not mean that all driving has to cease. Remember, I said a *single* occurrence. After all, don't we all have a misstep on our journeys now and then? As the caregiver, *do not overreact.* You will make yourself, and everyone concerned, a little crazy if you overdo it.

The Hartford Financial Services Group, Inc., in collaboration with the MIT Age Lab and Connecticut Community Care, Inc., (Couper, D., et al. 1999) conducted in-depth interviews with caregivers and people with dementia to learn how such families perceive and manage driving and transportation issues. The study was initiated because most information about dementia warns against driving, but does not describe how individuals and caregivers can determine when to stop.

How can you tell when it is time for a person to stop driving? The Hartford Study suggests: The decision to continue or stop driving needs to be based on a number of observations (listed below) and continuing discussions with the person with dementia, medical providers and caregivers. Those who have the ability to continue driving can reduce their risks by driving only on familiar roads, driving shorter distances and on less traveled roads, driving during daytime hours only, and avoiding rush hour traffic and bad weather driving.

Early warning signs of driving problems include:

- Incorrect signaling
- Trouble navigating turns
- Driving in the wrong lane
- Confusion at exits
- Parking inappropriately
- Hitting curbs
- Driving at inappropriate speeds
- Delayed responses to unexpected situations
- Not anticipating dangerous situations
- Increased agitation or irritation when driving
- Scrapes or dents on car, garage, or mailbox
- Getting lost in familiar places
- Near misses, ticketed moving violations, or warnings
- Car accident
- Confusing the brake and gas pedals
- Stopping in traffic for no apparent reason

Psychological changes in older adults can be due to the onset of dementia, Alzheimer's disease, or depression. An individual's reasoning ability can be greatly hampered as a result of any of these diseases. If seniors have been diagnosed with early signs of dementia or Alzheimer's disease, and have *not* demonstrated catastrophic driving habits, reducing their driving a little at a time is a better alternative than stopping them "cold turkey." If there has not been cause for an immediate need for the "tough-love" intervention of taking away the keys, then reduced time behind the wheel makes for a better transition. Some individuals diagnosed with early stage dementia can continue to drive, according to the Hartford study.

*Got Guilt?* The guilt we suffer when we must convince a parent to stop driving is complex. Our burden of guilt comes with the acknowledgment that we are dealing with a parent who has become two different people named *Then* and *Now*.

It is one more move to cut off another tentacle of that octopus we call independence. Our guilt becomes a vestige of remorse, and has the potential to overwhelm us. It frightens us as we acknowledge that taking away our parent's driving privileges adds another foggy layer to the lens we use to view our childhood memories. Through that lens, the images are a little less clear of the parent who took us on a dangerous yet fun adventure on a toboggan pulled slowly behind the car on a snowy deserted street. It fogs the childhood snapshot of a mom who was the first to volunteer for carpooling, Girl Scout outings, and impromptu drives to the Dairy Queen.

Another thought about guilt has to do with *who* is making you feel guilty? Are you bringing the guilt on yourself, or is it coming from another family member? Rev. Dr. James W. Ellor, who is a licensed clinical social worker and director of the Institute for Gerontology at Baylor University, counsels many families about dealing with elderly loved ones and dementia: "It is well documented that some seniors tend to manipulate their children, and if guilt helps, then it will get used. In this case, setting boundaries and helping the senior to understand one's own 'big picture' is often helpful."

**What Can You Do *Right Now*?** *Start the Conversation* Remember this affirmation in *every* discussion you have about reducing a parent's driving or stopping it completely. *Giving in Doesn't Mean Giving Up.* In other words, all independence is not lost because he or she has agreed to take public transportation or share rides with friends. It isn't a death sentence. But, the alternative, of driving while (age-) impaired could be.

In some cases, you can team up with seniors and have them help with the decision. Make a deal with an aging parent that together you will sell the car and use the money to provide transportation, i.e., a chauffeur, taxi-cab rides, or public transportation. See more about interventions near the end of this chapter in Action Steps.

Dr. Ellor suggests, "The big thing in my experience is not how fast to stop the driving, but rather how to help the parent remain functional. Many families try to take away the car, but then forget that Mom or Dad still needs to get out to go grocery shopping or to see friends, etc. The only way to be successful in removing driving is to remove the *need* for driving by arranging for alternatives. Then it can happen."

Some Good News

*When Renee, 87, visited her doctor for the first time after her extensive surgery, a 4-week hospital stay and 2 weeks in a rehab facility, she was overwhelmed by her doctor's good news. "After a good check-up, my doctor said, 'Now I want you to start driving.' I was so shocked. My doctor went on to explain, 'I know how much you were driving before, and how much you love it. If you don't start now, you will never go back to it.' I was thrilled."*

### How To Start the Communication

- Discuss driving tips you have read and those that are beneficial to you. This discussion may open a dialogue that your parent may want to have. "Yes, I've been worried about making left-hand turns too, especially at intersections where there is no 'left-turn' arrow."
- Keep a written record of your senior's driving incidents. (See Safe Driving Form at the end of this chapter.)
- Create opportunities to observe the driving habits of the person in question.
- Bring it back to the person in question.
  - Give examples of other crises, either involving someone dear to you who has been in an accident, or a traffic-accident story in the local paper.
  - It's time for *you* to renew your license.

**Not up for this Task?** If you feel you can't handle this task and discussion, call in the reinforcements. Get outside help. As Charlotte, 91, advised after she gave up driving a year earlier, "Find someone to intercede. If they [the parents] are not well, they are not thinking straight."

Find someone who is not connected by family ties and who can be openly objective. Here are a number of examples:

- Clergy
- Senior's peer or neighbor
- Physician
- Lawyers
- Therapist
- Care managers

**"The Doctor Said So"** The Depression Era generation revered family doctors as specialists, experts, and part of the family. Family doctors were respected. You can attempt to re-create the "family doc" relationship. Call the doctor before a visit and have a private conversation about your concerns. You may get blindsided by the physician about your parent's privacy because of the new confidentiality laws, but call anyway.

Many care receivers will take a directive from their physician more easily than from a family member or a friend. If the doctor says, "I would like you to not drive anymore," *and* writes it out on a prescription sheet, there's a good possibility that your senior will follow doctor's orders. Have the doctor prescribe a vision, hearing, and neurological exam.

When considering help from a physician:

- Seek out a geriatrician instead of a general practitioner. Due to the nature of his or her practice, the geriatrician will be more current on illnesses that cause changes in an elderly person's reaction time, vision, and on the side effects of medication prescribed for older adults.
- Check out vision programs. Go directly to an ophthalmologist or optometrist for vision testing.
- Have a private conversation with the doctor before the action. Let the physician hear your concerns and then assess your patient's physical condition and reaction skills.

What if you *still* meet with resistance?

- Continue anyway.
- Choose another direction.
- Get outside help (as suggested above).

**Take Someone Else for a Ride** Older drivers greatly reduced their risk of being involved in a fatal car crash when they were accompanied by at least one passenger in their car, according to research by Judith Geyer of the University of California, Berkeley. Reporting on research she presented at the 131st annual meeting of the American Public Health Association, of roughly 45,000 drivers in 2001 who had been in fatal crashes, male drivers 65 years and older reduced the risk of fatal crash by 20% when a passenger was in the car. If the driver was 85 years and older, the risk for the male drivers was reduced by 24%. According to Geyer, males driving alone had a crash rate nine times higher than with a passenger.

For female drivers aged 65 years and older, the risk of a fatal crash was reduced by 12% when a passenger was along for the ride. These statistics would certainly make one think twice about *not* leaving the "back-seat driver" at home.

Are you, as the adult child and caregiver, liable for your parent's car crash? No. You are not liable. (I can only assume that if we, as the adult children, were liable, interventions would happen at a much faster rate). According to legal counsel, adult children are not responsible if their parent becomes involved in a car crash. The *exception,* which should be common sense, is if an adult child lent his or her own car to a driver who was impaired. The impairment could be at any level including driving under the influence of alcohol, drugs, or disease or deterioration causing a lapse in judgment or skills.

The following is a "mini-series" of my dad's lifelong driving journey. As you get to know his character, you'll see how, with even the best intentions, love can make us lose our sense of direction.

*King of the Road: Part I*

> Note: My dad was a kind and loving man with his own set of
> eccentricities. I am sure many of you have a dad with similar charac-
> teristics. I would love to hear from you. (kconnect@rcn.com)

When it came to driving, Dad was King of the Road. Before World War II, he and his brother, Paul, started the Safeway Driving School. Who would have known that 45 years later, his kids would learn one of life's hard lessons in trying to get Dad to stop driving? It was his independence. It was his life.

Safeway Driving School had a huge fleet of cars, and Dad and my uncle Paul had many, many customers. This was in the '40s, long before Drivers Education was introduced through the schools. Our family was an exception to the one-car-per-household norm in the 1950s, because there was always a driving school car at my dad's disposal in addition to the family car.

One of Dad's later-to-become-famous driving students was Nancy Davis, who later became Mrs. Ronald Reagan. Dad cherished Nancy Reagan as his pupil, and kept in touch with her through notes well into his 70s. He even had an autographed picture of her, which she had sent, posted on his dresser mirror.

Because he was a driving instructor, it was my dad who taught my mom and each of his three kids to drive. He and my mom took the driving instruction very seriously, and presented an even bigger challenge to each of us regarding getting our driver's licenses: we had to be tested while driving a car with a manual transmission. For any of our readers who get an instant panic attack thinking about that mantra of, "First gear, clutch, brake; second gear, clutch, brake; and third gear, brake, clutch," your worst fears were realized. We also had to exhibit expert parking skills by being able to demonstrate parallel parking uphill. In hindsight, my parents' promise that, having mastered the manual transmission shifting skill, we would be able to drive anything, was true. Now, any Jeep, truck, Humvee, or rental car that comes equipped with a manual transmission is ready for our expertise.

My dad started his driving adventures in a small Indiana town, where everyone on the roads knew where you were going. He continued to drive on the busy city streets of Chicago as if he were still navigating the terrain in a small town. Why use directional signals? Everyone knew where he was going, so why let them know he was turning left?

The other piece of this puzzle that fueled his buildup to bad driving habits came indirectly from my mother. Throughout most of their 57 years of marriage, my mom was the manager, the financial wizard, and navigator, which meant that she read the road maps and knew the directions. In short, she told my dad where to go. He had very little sense of direction. She led, he followed. The unhappy result of one of their unsuccessful excursions in later life is profiled in King of the Road: Part V section in this chapter.

### King of the Road: Part II

The driving troubles began long before Dad was a danger to himself and others on the road. Like a tumor the size of a pinhead, these incidents seemed small and insignificant at the time. Now, in hindsight, because we are smarter and the roads are more dangerous, those small incidents could have added up to a deadly malignancy. Take seat belts, for example. When seat belts were first introduced in the '60s, Dad saw no significant reason to have them, so he cut them out of any car he purchased.

### An Obstinate King of the Road: Part III

*Early Warning Signs*  We continued to be a two-car family even after my father closed down the driving school. In early 1960, Dad purchased a truck for his new business, leaving Mom with the family car. When she started to work outside the home as a part-time church secretary and their jobs were in opposite directions, two cars were still a necessity.

Because money was tight, more often than not my parents were both driving old cars that needed frequent repairs. In the mid-80s, with all of the kids now into adulthood and living independently, my parents were empty nesters—two people driving two old clunker vehicles badly in need of costly repairs.

My brother, sister, and I wanted to make this situation better, and together bought Mom and Dad a used station wagon that had very few miles on the odometer, and was in excellent condition. Besides providing my folks with a safe car, this move would be financially beneficial to them. They would be driving one good car that would require little maintenance, and they would not be financially supporting two cars with insurance, repairs, and state and city vehicle licenses and registration.

It was a perfect plan—except for one snag. My dad wanted his own car. He fiercely guarded his independence, and he possessed a childlike bad habit of not wanting to share. Tensions between my parents mounted during the first few months of this single-car-family arrangement because my dad didn't like adjusting his plans around the use of the car. Who suffered? My mom. More often than not, she ended up taking public transportation when a compromise about use of the car couldn't be reached.

Accustomed to getting his way, my dad pushed the envelope and made an emotional family volcano erupt when he went out and purchased a second car on the sly. To make matters worse, it was a clunker … not fit for driving. My dad answered a for-sale ad in the local paper, and purchased a 15-year-old Ford Mustang from a 19-year-old stranger for $400. To add insult to injury, over the next 15 months my dad poured $2,000 into repairs for the Mustang. That money came out of a very sparse family budget that had no cushion for repair costs of this kind. But, what cost our family much more than the dollars spent on the Ford Mustang was the emotional disharmony that erupted as a result of my dad's selfish act.

Could we have stopped dad from purchasing the second car? Was there another alternative to getting a second car? Could a third party, other than a family member, have helped with the discord that resulted from my dad's purchase? Take a hard look at the Action Steps near the end of this chapter.

### King of the Road: Part IV

*Bucking the System*    At age 70-something, Dad went for his driving test, failed the behind-the-wheel portion, and then chewed out the young driving instructor. Not to be defeated, he scooped up his paperwork, and drove to the next drivers' testing facility a few miles away, where he passed with flying colors and they renewed his license. He then wrote a scathing letter to the Illinois Secretary of State, letting him know what imbeciles he had encountered at the testing facility where he had failed his test. This was my dad. He was ornery, obstinate, a great innovator, a renegade, and a free spirit. This was my father, who 50 years earlier had owned and managed one of the most successful driving schools in the city of Chicago.

### King of the Road: Part V

*Warning Signs and Stupid Mistakes*    It was 1993, at the time when my mother had been diagnosed with early stage Alzheimer's disease. She had given up driving with ease at the suggestion of her doctor. Now, Dad was the official chauffeur, even though, by this time, we had seen and shrugged off various warning signs that he, too, should not have been behind the wheel. I was at work that day in my role as executive director of a retirement facility in Chicago. It was noon, and I was having lunch in the resident dining room with some prospective residents.

The receptionist of the facility came into the dining room to let me know that my father was on the phone and wanted to speak with me. Thinking there wasn't a sense of urgency, and wanting to seal the deal with these prospective clients, I asked if I could possibly call him back.

Our receptionist, Marilyn, bent down and whispered into my ear that she thought I ought to take this call. She said, "Your mom and dad are driving in Oak Lawn [Chicago suburb], and your dad is lost."

I excused myself, answered the call, and put a face on the body of the story that was rapidly unfolding from my dad, who was calling from a phone booth. This was in a decade long before Onstar navigation systems and cell phones. In hindsight, my old-fashioned dad would probably not have used either one anyway, even if he had them. Even if they were free.

The scenario was one that had happened before. But what had changed was the mental capacity of the players. All their married lives Mom had been the navigator. She knew the directions and the addresses of their many destinations. My mom told my dad how to get there and he followed her lead.

On this particular day, my mom knew she had a doctor's appointment at 2 o'clock in Oak Lawn. What was different today, however, was that she couldn't retrieve any information from her brain as to the exact address of the doctor's office, a location she had been to dozens of times before. She couldn't even recall the major cross streets. For the majority of her previous visits to the doctor, she had driven herself.

As my dad poured out their dilemma, I ran this video through my head. For today's appointment, she had told my dad that they needed to be in Oak Lawn for the appointment at 2 o'clock. He complied, and they journeyed out with true destination unknown. Once lost, he was calling for help. Not to be too stereotypical, but my dad fit the mold of "men who don't ask for directions," and rarely asked for help.

Because I knew that my dad *did* possess an innate knowledge of architect and city planner Daniel Burnham's street grid system of Chicago, where all the streets run in 8-block miles by numbers, I knew that I could redirect my dad toward home. I put on my imaginary flight-controller cap and found out his exact location by having him identify the cross streets outside the phone booth. And like a flight controller talks an airplane down through the dense fog, I was able to talk my dad through how to get to Cicero Avenue by way of landmarks, and navigate his way home. God smiled on this whole scenario because fortunately, I was familiar with the area where they had become lost. They made it home, frustrated, tired, embarrassed, and having missed the doctor's appointment. But they were safe.

Could this episode have been prevented? Had I and my siblings witnessed and ignored various warning signs? Absolutely. Would our intervention have taken away some of their independence, which was now so precious? Probably. Had my family and I been proactive, been armed with, and put into gear some preventive action steps, this episode could have been avoided.

*Still in the Driver's Seat*

> *The same year Ralph turned 88, he had bypass surgery on his heart and didn't like temporarily giving up driving, even for the month of his recovery. Back behind the wheel today, he is restricted on his driver's license to drive only during daylight hours because of his eyesight. His ophthalmologist conducted the vision test. Ralph says, "Not driving at night is a lot better now since the time has switched to Daylight Savings Time, but the biggest hang-up is when it gets dark early during the winter, and you can't linger a little longer if you want to. You have to get home before dark.*
>
> *"I dread the thought; I'm not denying that. I think about it. When the time comes and I can't drive anymore. There are so many little things you want to get out and do. You want something from the store.*
>
> *"When I was laid up after my surgery, my daughters would do the shopping. But there is always something you forget to tell them to get. Sometimes they buy things that are not to your liking.*
>
> *"I don't like to be dependent on anyone. When the time comes, I guess I will have to do a lot more planning with activities. I fully realize the time will come."*
>
> **—Ralph, 88, living in a suburb of Chicago**

## What to Do About It

*Action Steps*

- Set up an account with a taxi service so that the impaired person doesn't have to worry about paying for a ride. For those nieces and nephews who don't have a clue what to buy their elderly uncles for holiday gifts, suggest some taxi vouchers.
- Find out what kinds of services your city bus service has for seniors and the handicapped.

- Call the local churches and find out about volunteers who will drive people around town to do errands.
- Move your person to an area that provides better transportation. Did I say *move?* Isn't moving a better alternative than to have an elderly care receiver isolated and feeling deprived because his or her set of wheels is gone?
- Do the reverse-commute idea with local vendors. Not only can you get just about anything delivered these days, there are podiatrists, hair stylists and bankers who make house calls. If vendors want to keep long time-customers happy and retain their business, they will do whatever it takes to bring their services to you. (If you don't really believe this, our veterinarian brought our family dog back to my home after a visit when an emergency business meeting at my home office kept me from being able to pick up my pet.) Sometimes, all you have to do is ask.
- Visits from friends could include outings; for example, going to a movie and stopping at a grocery store along the way. A lot of restaurants and movie theaters offer senior discounts during the daylight hours when it is safer to be out and to drive.

*Where to Turn for Help*   The *55 Alive AARP Driver Safety Program* is the nation's first and largest classroom driver-refresher course specially designed for motorists aged 50 and up. It is intended to help older drivers improve their skills while teaching them to avoid accidents and traffic violations.

Call the AARP main number to find out information about driving programs in your state: 1-888-687-2277. Or contact AARP at 601 E. Street NW, Washington, DC 20049/ www.aarp.org/55 alive

**Auto Insurance Discounts**   Drivers who have completed the AARP Driver Safety Program are eligible for auto-insurance discounts in some states. Upon completing the 8-hour program, the driver receives a course-completion certificate that can then be presented to his or her insurance agent. Depending on the state in which the driver lives and the insurance company's policies, he or she may be eligible for an automobile insurance-premium reduction or discount that can be received in one of two ways: (1) the driver is a resident of a state that mandates a discount for anyone completing an approved driver refresher course, or (2) the automobile insurance company voluntarily offers a discount.

To ascertain which states now have a law that mandates an automobile insurance discount for anyone completing an approved driver-improvement course, call your local Secretary of State's office.

The Department of Health and Human Services aims to reduce motor vehicle-related deaths among people of all ages to no more than 12 per 100,000 people by 2010. For adults older than age 70, the motor vehicle death rate has remained stable at about 23 per 100,000 for over a decade (Department of Health and Human Services 2000).

*Tips To Discuss with Your Family Member*   Here's a handy form distributed by the people of The Hartford. I think its purpose is a good one, and that's why I have included it here. But, I can bet you dollars to donuts that family members who have mild dementia will not fill this out. Would you if you were in their shoes? Would you rat yourself out to your adult daughter that you've become lost, moved inappropriately into the wrong lane and hit a few curbs? I don't think so.

*The Hartford: "At the Crossroads—A Guide to Alzheimer's Disease, Dementia & Driving"*

Warning Signs for Drivers with Dementia

Have you noticed any of the following warning signs?
Is there a change in the number or frequency of these warning signs?
Do the circumstances and seriousness of the warning signs warrant continued close monitoring, driving modifications or an immediate end to driving?

| Warning Signs | Date(s) | Notes (Severity/Frequency) |
|---|---|---|
| Incorrect signaling | | |
| Trouble navigating turns | | |
| Moving into a wrong lane | | |
| Confusion at exits | | |
| Parking inappropriately | | |
| Hitting curbs | | |
| Driving at inappropriate speeds | | |
| Delayed responses to unexpected situations | | |
| Not anticipating potential dangerous situations | | |
| Increased agitation or irritation when driving | | |
| Scrapes or dents on the car, garage, or mailbox | | |
| Getting lost in familiar places | | |
| Near misses | | |
| Ticketed moving violations or warnings | | |
| Car accident | | |
| Confusing brake and gas pedals | | |

Stopping in traffic for no apparent reason_____
Other signs: _____
(©2000 The Hartford. Reprinted with permission.)

For the complete brochure from The Hartford, go to www.thehart-ford.com/alzheimers/brochure.

You can also request brochures by writing to:

The Hartford
At the Crossroads
200 Executive Boulevard
Southington, CT 06489

*Family Agreement Form*

This form is for you, the empowered caregiver

*Think of it as a report card.* It is to help you to record every single instance of your mom's saying that people drive too fast, or that she knew she drove past the beauty shop three different times. If your elderly uncle has had one fender bender too many, and you know about them, *record every detail.* In the worst possible scenarios, you don't want to be caught in a crisis situation where there has been a bad accident, and you recall that, "Now that I think about it, he did say several times that he missed the same exits he has been using all his life."

Using this form, (and when I say "using" I mean really filling it out), could provide you with evidence to present to a physician when you need to stack the deck with a professional to get an elderly person to stop driving.

Agreement with My Family about Driving

To my family:

*The time may come when I can no longer make the best decisions for the safety of others and myself. Therefore, in order to help my family make necessary decisions, this statement is an expression of my wishes and directions while I am still able to make these decisions. I have discussed with my family my desire to drive as long as it is safe for me to do so.*

*When it is not reasonable for me to drive, I desire _____ (person's name) to tell me I can no longer drive. I trust my family will take the necessary steps to prohibit my driving in order to ensure my safety and the safety of others while protecting my dignity.*

Signed_____ Date _____
Copies of this request have been shared with: _____
(©2000 The Hartford. Reprinted with permission.)

*Skills Review Courses*  Most states offer a Rules of the Road review course. Contact your local Secretary of State's office to find out times and dates. In Illinois, the free class is offered 3,000 times a year in 600 locations statewide. You can find your Secretary of State's Web site at www.Secretaryofstate.com.

**Other Great Resources**  *AAA Foundation for Traffic Safety.* Lots of information about supplemental transportation for seniors. Publications, guides for families, and a self-exam.
www.seniordrivers.org
www.Aaafts.org

AAA Foundation for Traffic Safety
Administrative Office
607 14th Street NW
Washington, DC 20005
800-305-7233
Tel: 202-638-5944
Fax: 202-638-5943

Safe Senior Driving: A consumer-friendly website about safe senior citizen driving: www.helpguide.org

*The Road Ahead*

Your parent's safety and happiness are the highest priorities. By using the resources outlined here and your own personal rules of the road fueled by love and compassion, your journey through this process will take both of you to a happy, and mishap-free destination.

# CHAPTER 8

# Leaving Home

## When Your Elderly Parent Must Move

*You take a tree from it roots, and the tree dies.*

> —Helen, 86, grew up, raised her family, and grew old
> in Philadelphia. Two years ago, against her wishes,
> she moved to Florida to be closer to her son.

Moving away from the home that you love, from all that is comfortable and familiar, takes on a whole new meaning when a medical condition or frailty forces you out. Elderly individuals—many of whom have been adamant about keeping their independence—are faced with this predicament every day. It's a tough situation to be in, especially if the decision has been made for you, not by you, and if you've lived in your own home for several decades.

Imagine yourself in the above scenario. Wouldn't you feel a terrible sense of loss? Now, to add insult to injury, imagine having to give up valued possessions because your new living space is too small to accommodate them. Doesn't this compound your sense of loss? You will surely agree that this downsizing of space and dispersion of cherished items—both voluntary and involuntary—is a depressing proposition.

Adult children or caregivers should do everything possible to include the aging parent in this decision. Before you uproot your parent from his or her own home, please explore every option. But if you, together, decide that such a move is the best option, don't agonize over it. Moving from the family home into a new housing situation—i.e., a retirement community or nursing home, or even into your home (see Chapter 9)—shouldn't be seen as a defeat. Ideally, the move is in the best interest of the elderly individual, intended to enhance his or her quality of life.

If the move is inevitable, an action plan designed by both the displaced senior and the caregiver will help both parties deal with the downsizing process.

### Fear of the Unknown

Most of us don't like change, and the elderly are no exception. As children, we feared the unknown in new schools, in our first day at camp, in the process of making new friends. Individuals who have had to move to age-segregated housing—whether it is a retirement facility, congregate home, or nursing home—experience the same fears about their new surroundings.

*"What if I can't find the dining room?"*
*"Can I bring my own furniture?"*
*"Why am I living with strangers?"*
*"Can my cat live with me?"*

### The Resistance to Change

The dependent elderly, given a choice, would almost certainly not opt to live in a skilled nursing facility. Do you know any frail individuals who are the exception? Have you ever heard a senior whose health is failing say "I can't wait to give up most of my things, live in a smaller space, and move into a room with a stranger?" Ask anyone over the age of 80 his or her perception of a nursing home and you'll get, "It's 'the old folks home.'" When my father became an octogenarian and his health started to fail, he would not entertain the idea of he and my mother moving into a retirement-living community, let alone assisted living or a nursing home. His ubiquitous lament? "It's full of old people."

### Making the Move—Setting the Wheels in Motion

*Downsizing*    The generation that is being displaced is made up of individuals from the Depression era, who were taught to save tinfoil, to return milk bottles for deposit refunds, to crochet pillowcases and handkerchiefs. They have had to grow into being part of the "throw-away" society. It is not surprising that these people resist "throwing away" their treasured possessions.

Some individuals have to give up beloved pets. For older women, who have to give up handmade items and antiques that won't fit into their new, smaller apartments, the change can be traumatic. Older men suffer as well. Many men raised their families in homes that had a basement full of tools and a workbench. Others had garages stocked with automotive and lawn care supplies. Men of this generation fixed lawnmowers and motors and gadgets. The loss of their space and tools is upsetting, indeed.

> *Heck, yes, it was tough to give up our house. We had to sell or give away a lot. We wish we could be back in our house every day, but my wife couldn't climb the stairs to the bathroom. I couldn't handle the upkeep anymore. What I miss most … is the house."*
>
> **—Paul (pseudonym), 87, and his wife moved to a retirement facility 10 years ago after living in their former home for 30 years. His wife died last year.**

### Distribution of Treasures

Having to give away or sell sentimental possessions is a large, emotional part of downsizing. It is critical that the dependent adult be a partner in the dissolution of personal property. No one should be "dictated to" at such a sensitive time in his or her life.

*Sentimental Value:* If the individual who is moving has heirlooms, jewelry that won't be worn, or items that have a personal meaning or rich family heritage, he or she should pass them on now. In many ways, this is far preferable to "willing" such items. The giver will enjoy seeing nieces or grandchildren appreciate and enjoy their treasures. In many families, cherished pieces of china or jewelry are given as gifts at holiday time or birthdays.

*Garage or yard sales:* If the dispersal of personal items will take place at neighborhood sales, dependent elderly people should be present, if possible. If haggling over prices is a practice at the sale, let them be involved in the bartering or set the pricing. This will give them a greater sense of control.

*Items for Charity:* Try to have the person who is donating the items present at the drop-off, and follow up with a personal note to the charity with the donor's name. Suggest that the charity send a personal thank-you card along with a reference as to how the items will be used. Suggest that a personal history of the item be either written out or told to an administrator of the charity, so that the story of its heritage can be passed on.

### Is This a Mistake?

*Possible Alternatives to Moving* As mentioned earlier, you should do everything possible to include your aging parent in the decision. If you are certain that a move is best, come up with concrete evidence for discussion. And before you make a final decision, make you sure you have explored every option for keeping your parent in his or her familiar home.

*Adult Day Care*

The majority of adult day care programs are community based, offering the frail elderly supervised programs and meals for a full or partial day. Programs are geared toward individuals who are functional or only cognitively impaired. Some day care centers provide transportation. Payment plans are available with some payment offered on a sliding scale. Senior centers, local area agencies on aging, and disease-specific organizations such as the National Alzheimer's Disease Association have information about adult day care programs.

Sometimes Timing is Everything

*During World War II, Cathy was chief bacteriologist at the 700-bed Roosevelt Hospital in New York. One of her most prominent patients during her tenure was Madame Chiang, wife of Chiang Kai-Shek, the former ruler of mainland China. With a strong Italian heritage, Cathy speaks Italian fluently, and understands every word of the lyric opera without having to read the English subtitles, according to her husband Herb.*

*Cathy, 89, was diagnosed with Alzheimer's disease in 1998. Cathy's mother had Alzheimer's also, so she knew what lay ahead. When she first learned of her diagnosis, Cathy suggested to Herb that he divorce her, because she knew her need for care would use up all their assets. Herb refused. He loved her too much. "We did wait too long to get long-term-care insurance," he admits, adding that he has a policy, but that Cathy was denied because of her Alzheimer's diagnosis.*

*Although she is still able to live at home in Chicago, Cathy attends adult day care 3 days a week through a program at the Council for Jewish Elderly. A caregiver comes in daily to be with Cathy when Herb isn't home and to do household chores.*

*When Cathy and Herb first went to check out the adult day care program several years ago, Cathy took one look around and said, "I'm not ready for this." Two years have gone by and her disease has progressed. Now Cathy enjoys her time at the day-care center. "The people [at the day care center] are very nice," she says. "We have a lot of programs—entertainment, activities, crafts. But I'm happiest with Herbie."*

*Respite Care*

Many long-term care facilities and adult day care programs offer respite care, a temporary short-term stay where care and meals are included. Some nursing homes and assisted-living facilities offer respite stays as a "trial run" for individuals who are considering full time residency. The respite programs are a benefit for family members who must travel out of town and are unable to take their elderly parent along, or those who are unable to bring in additional help at home. Information about respite programs can be obtained by calling local long-term care facilities.

### Hiring In-Home Help

*Home Care: Hiring Through an Agency*   Home care workers provide non-skilled services or custodial care, such as help with a person's activities of daily living (ADLs). These include bathing, dressing, toileting, transferring, grooming, and ambulation. Many home care agencies also provide staff to do light housekeeping and chore work. A list of questions to ask the agency is included at the end of this chapter.

*Hiring an Independent Caregiver*   When hiring a caregiver who works independently and is not affiliated with an agency there are many issues to consider and questions to ask. Many referrals for caregivers come by word of mouth, through churches, or local senior-service agencies. Your local Area Agency on Aging will give you referrals for qualified caregivers. A list of questions and considerations about hiring an independent home-care worker is included at the end of this chapter.

> *At 91, Lucille (pseudonym) is fiercely independent. Several years ago, when she had been hospitalized for a short time, she found herself suddenly reliant on others. "I accepted care because it was necessary," she says. Should she require additional care in the future, she would like a say about who provides it and how her care is handled. "I would like a person who is a sympathetic person, not bossy. Someone who could sympathize with my problems."*

### What's Out There?

*Independent Living*   Called retirement living, this option provides residents with their own private apartment. They can usually bring their own furnishings. Meals, transportation, and activities are included in the monthly fee. Payment plans vary. Sometimes rent is paid monthly; other times an endowment is paid up front with a monthly fee collected thereafter.

*Continuing Care Retirement Communities (CCRC)*   A CCRC offers a long-term care contract that provides for the continuum of care through the end of the resident's life. Residents transition through the community of services as their health declines. Service offerings usually include independent living, assisted living, additional home-care services and skilled nursing home care. Endowment and nominal monthly fee are typical.

*Assisted-Living Facility*    Representing the middle tier between independent living and skilled nursing care, assisted living is geared to individuals
who can no longer live independently, but who don't require the care of a
nurse. Assisted-living units—usually rooms and apartments—are smaller
than their independent counterparts. A la carte services are usually available. Onsite home-care personnel can be hired to escort residents to meals,
to provide morning and evening care, and to assist with activities of daily
living.

Assisted living costs average about $30,864 annually. The most expen-
sive assisted facility in the country, in Stamford, Connecticut, averages
about $52,000 per year. The least expensive is in Miami, Florida at $16,000
per year. Increases per year average about 6%.

> *Two 91-year-old women, living in different cities in Wisconsin,*
> *made the transition to a nursing home and a retirement community,*
> *respectively. They offer completely different perspectives on their new*
> *living arrangements.*
>
> *When Rose, a widow who lived alone, experienced some physical*
> *difficulties and had trouble taking care of her house, she spoke to her*
> *adult children about moving to a nursing home. "I said, 'Somebody's*
> *got to take care of me', because [my daughter] Fran worked, [my son]*
> *Ron worked, and my other son's working. I am not so feeble that I*
> *don't realize they have to make a living just like I do."*
>
> *Rose moved into a nursing home just outside of Lake Geneva, Wis-*
> *consin, stayed 5 days, and moved back home. "I thought I didn't need*
> *this yet. I wasn't ready for it. They're not really giving you everything*
> *[doing everything for you] like a box with a ribbon tied around it. I*
> *thought, 'I can still cook for myself.' In other words, you're really fool-*
> *ing yourself. You think you can do more than you can. You slow*
> *down."*
>
> *Once home and alone, Rose looked around her kitchen and became*
> *frightened. She feared she would fall, or become faint and be unable to*
> *get help.*
>
> *Rose returned to the nursing home after 5 days at home. "The*
> *young girls here, the aides, they treat me well. They say ' Hi Rosie,*
> *how are you doing?' and that makes me feel good."*
>
> *Side note: When Rose and I met in her room at the nursing home*
> *where she lives, we had to close the door because of the loud commo-*
> *tion coming from down the hall. The home's pet mynah bird was pro-*
> *ducing all the noise as it squawked "Nurse! Nurse! Nurse!" We could*
> *barely hear ourselves talk. Clearly, although Rose has moved on to*

*what will probably be her final residence, her adventures in her new
spirited environment continue.*

Assisted Living—Not for Everyone

*Lucille and her husband Clyde (pseudonyms) live in an urban area
of Wisconsin. Although they have lived in their current home for 12
years, they took a brief hiatus and moved to an assisted-living community when her husband broke his hip. As soon as it was healed, they
moved back home. "I couldn't stand it," Lucille says. "We were talked
into moving to assisted living by my children. We had a nice apartment,
three rooms. I moved a lot of furniture in, while our house stood empty."*

*After her husband went through physical therapy, Lucille contin-
ued her campaign to move home. 'Why in the world can't we move
[back] there?' I would say." The couple stayed at the assisted living
facility for 1 year. "It seemed like forever."*

*Lucille's biggest disappointments were with the service and the
socialization of the other residents. "It was hit or miss. We didn't
really know what we were getting into. You really don't have any
freedom of your own. We like to eat when we are ready." It was also
difficult to make new friends, according to Lucille. "You couldn't get
anyone to play cards. They all stayed in their apartments. You are in
with a bunch of strangers. It takes a long time to develop good
friendships."*

*At 91, Lucille continues to drive and plays cards once a week with
several of her friends. She and her husband are back, and happy, in
their own home.*

*Assisted Living on the High Seas*    In a study published by the American
Geriatrics Society, physicians Lee A. Lindquist and Robert M. Golub
(2004) compared amenities, costs, and services provided by assisted living
facilities and those offered by luxury cruise lines. Their findings revealed
that over a 20-year life expectancy after moving to an assisted living facility, nursing home, or cruise ship, the quality of services was superior on
the cruise ship. Dr. Lindquist also found that the net costs of cruise ship
living were only about $2,000 higher than those associated with assisted
living facilities over the 20-year period.

Dr. Lindquist, an instructor of medicine at Northwestern University
Feinberg School of Medicine said, "A cruise ship could be considered a
floating assisted living facility, offering many amenities, such as three
meals a day with escorts to meals, physicians on site and housekeeping and
laundry services. The research also revealed that the employee to-customer
ratio on a cruise ship far outnumbered those staff in the assisted living

facilities. The largest cruise lines—Royal Caribbean, Holland America, Celebrity, and Norwegian Cruise Lines— average a ratio of two or three passengers per employee. Nursing home and assisted living employees are each responsible for significantly more patients, according to the report.

Other advantages to the extended cruise ship living for seniors included 24-hour physician and nurse availability, changing scenery daily, and the sociability of the elderly interacting with the regular passengers.

Assisted living programs aboard cruise ships are only in the concept stage. None of the cruise lines offer such services or programs yet. If such assisted living packages could be implemented, continuous cruise ship living would offer elderly individuals a luxurious global travel alternative to existing senior housing. Bon voyage!

*Skilled Nursing Facility* Nursing homes are licensed by the state, with requirements set by regulatory commissions. Patients are the very sick or those who need rehab. Most offer short rehabilitation stays, respite care, and Medicare-covered recovery stays. Some provide hospice services. Financial coverage includes Medicare, state aid and coverage by various health insurance policies. There is a day rate for room and board. Medication and many of the services have additional costs.

*Understaffing: Who's Minding the Store?* A universal problem in long-term care facilities is understaffing. Although facilities go to painstaking lengths to make sure the patient-to-staff ratio is sufficient, call-offs and high turnover consistently strain the work force. Night shifts, weekends, and holidays are the hardest hit.

Dorothy, a 90-year-old resident of a nursing facility in the Chicago suburbs, told about a particular Valentine's Day that fell on a Saturday. "You could have thrown a football down the hall that day and not hit a soul," she says. "Everyone called in sick so that they could enjoy their Valentine's Day."

The best way for family members and caregivers to address such concerns is to be watchdogs and advocates. Let the administrator know your concerns, and ask how the problem is going to be rectified. If complaints fall on deaf ears, or if grievances are not addressed, go to state licensing agencies, the Joint Commission on Accreditation, or the local department of public health. Be the "squeaky wheel."

*Another Way To Be Heard* The Breakers at Edgewater Beach, a retirement community in Chicago that's part of Senior Lifestyle Corporation, takes a novel approach to encouraging residents and family members to voice their concerns, complaints, and compliments. At the front desk are small comment card brochures that bear the executive director's first name on the front panel. Below his name is the following checklist:

Hey Christopher!

- ☐ I'm dazzled!
- ☐ Pleasantly surprised
- ☐ Satisfied
- ☐ A bit annoyed
- ☐ Mad as heck
- ☐ I have a compliment
- ☐ I have a concern
- ☐ Here's why…

On the inside of the pamphlet, the resident or family member has the opportunity to write out concerns or complaints.

*Subsidized Senior Housing*    The federal government and most states have programs that help pay for housing for older people with low or moderate incomes. In most cases, these housing facilities are rental units. Because there is a very large segment of the population that qualifies for subsidized senior housing, there may be a waiting list. Advance planning is a must, as waiting lists can run from 7 to 10 years. If you find that your loved one "needs it now," his or her chances of being accepted are slim. Anticipate the need. If subsidized housing is the only way to go due to limited financial resources, it is imperative that you get on a waiting list years before your move has to take place.

Some of these housing programs also offer help with meals and other activities such as housekeeping, shopping, and doing the laundry. Usually a federal or state agency will review your monthly income and expenses to see if you are eligible for this type of housing.

Subsidized high-rise living is most commonly referred to as Section 202 housing by the federal government. Call your local area agency on aging or 800-677-1116 to find out about Section 202 housing in your area.

The federal Department of Housing and Urban Development (HUD) operates a special Web site (www.hud.gov/senior) regarding subsidized housing issues, or you can call HUD at 888-569-4287 for additional information.

*Location*    Take inventory regarding your aging parent's needs and desires. Should the move be to an independent setting, an assisted living facility, or a skilled nursing care facility? More importantly, what does the senior want to do? Is his view realistic? Does he want to be in an urban setting with transportation, close access to stores, the theater or the local hospital? Is a suburban or rural setting more appropriate with its wide-open spaces, ponds, and birds? Is proximity to her doctor a priority? Does she want to be closer to you?

*Let the Shopping Begin*    Shopping for a new place to live can be as challenging as actually moving in. Tours of senior living facilities by prospective residents or family members can be stressful, especially if a discharge from a hospital makes the need immediate. Every situation is different.

Having been on both sides of the tour—as the facility manager and as the adult daughter looking for a retirement apartment living and then a skilled nursing facility for my own parents—I know that this experience can be a walk in the park or completely unsettling. Many adult children who tour a long-term care facility don't know what to expect.

Touring nursing homes often proves to be very difficult for the family caregiver who has never been in this type of environment. It is not unusual for a family on tour to be met in the hallway by an irate resident who may say, "Get me out of here!" or, "I'm not supposed to be here. They've got the wrong guy!"

Remember that in the last four decades the profile of the "typical" nursing home patient has shifted. Hospitals used to keep the sick, frail elderly for days or even weeks after an operation or illness. With the onset of the Medicare Prospective Payment System (PPS), introduced by the federal government in October 1983, hospitals started getting paid a predetermined rate for each Medicare admission. Each patient is classified into a Diagnosis Related Group, (DRG) and the hospital is paid a flat rate regardless of the actual services provided. Patients are moved out of the hospitals at a rapid rate, with the result that the frail elderly now spend their days convalescing in skilled nursing homes.

Assisted living, the newest component to long-term care, brings an intermediate layer to the continuum of care arena. When frail individuals need help with mobility, bathing, dressing, and toileting— all ADLs —they are candidates for assisted living. Because individuals who qualify for the assisted living tier are no longer in "the old-folks home," today's nursing home residents remain the sickest patients and the ones who require continuous care from doctors and nurses.

Sometimes the best-laid plans for visiting facilities can go awry. A winning proposition for first-time visitors is to have done your homework and know what you are looking for. If this is your first experience in visiting a skilled nursing facility, don't be surprised to see elderly individuals who are very sick or out of sorts because of their situations. While you may encounter some residents who are full of cheer, remember that the majority of nursing-home patients live there because they are ill or convalescing, they are not there by choice. They are there to have a need fulfilled—to receive round-the-clock skilled nursing attention.

*Make the Shopping Trip a Success* **Action Steps** Know the right questions to ask. (An expanded list of questions about safety, meals, finances and services is included at the end of the chapter.)

- Ask to tour the kitchen.
- Ask for a reference list. This will include patients' families who have given their consent to be called as references for the facility.
- Find out what happens during an emergency.
- What part of the costs and fees are refundable?
- Although you may learn what the staff-to-patient ratio is, be prepared for a skeleton crew to be running the show on weekends and holidays.

## *It Doesn't Have To Be a Life Sentence—Is There an Escape Route?*

Even some television commercials portray seniors in nursing homes as trying to escape their confines. For example, there is a popular auto commercial about an elderly man escaping to go on an adventure to Las Vegas with his grandson. It depicts an elderly nursing home resident dressed to go out, complete with a tweed hat. He looks both ways to make sure the coast is clear as he leaves his room. He sneaks past the sleeping attendant at the nurses' station and gingerly creeps past the exercise class going through their paces in the day room.

Having given all of his attendants the slip, we see him emerge into the sunlight, and then spot a shiny new car parked across the street waiting to take him away. Behind the wheel is his grandson, who greets him with "Hey, Grandpop" to which he replies, "Hey, Bubba." The two speed off into the sunset in the car. The last two frames show the elderly gentleman flinging his hat out the sunroof as they pass a road sign that says "Las Vegas."

Such humor is a healthy way to deal with a resident's situation. We must realize that the mindset of escaping is not so much to leave the facility, but to escape from a physical body of declining health. Moving to a long-term care facility need not be viewed as a penal life sentence. A lot depends on the resident's state of mind. The health and happiness of each individual in a nursing home is directly related to his or her positive attitude. Overall, skilled nursing facilities provide caring, friendly environments, and a wide variety of quality services.

Individuals who previously led isolated lives and lacked socialization most often begin to thrive in their new nursing home settings with newly found friendships and a renewed sense of belonging. Rose, who was introduced earlier in this chapter, relished the attention she received from the nurses aides and other residents' family members. Much of the success and happiness of nursing home residents comes from within their own souls.

## Age-Segregated Living—A Matter of Choice

Some retirement communities have taken steps to appear intergenerational by housing preschool centers on the retirement campuses or offering learning classes where the elderly and young adults share classroom space. This type of environment offers the elderly an opportunity to stay current with the lifestyles of younger generations.

Living in a community of similar-aged people is not to everyone's liking. Reese Palley, the 70-something sailor and author of *Unlikely Passages* (1998), said of age-segregated living: "My generation must escape from the tyranny of the young and avoid relegation to those holding tanks for the truly old and decrepit."

## Resources and Information about Long Term Care

*Choosing a Long-Term Care Facility*   The following questions will be beneficial when searching for a facility:

1. Is there adequate staff-to-resident ratio?
2. What services are included in the monthly fee?
3. What if my parent wants additional services?
4. What if my parent requires more care than this facility provides?
5. What if there is a sudden change in my parent's medical condition?

*Accommodations*

1. Do you have guest accommodations?
2. How many residents share a bathroom?
3. Can residents bring their own furniture and personal effects to decorate?
4. Is the carpeting in the room or apartment replaced after every move-out?

*Administration*

1. Is there a resident council?
2. Is there a family council?
3. Is there a referral list of families who have loved ones in the facility?

*Safety*

1. What is the evacuation procedure in the event of fire, tornado, etc?
2. Is there security on duty 24 hours a day?
3. Is there a nurse on duty 24 hours a day, 7 days a week?

4. Are residents allowed to smoke in their apartment or room?
5. Does each unit have a sprinkler system and smoke detectors?
6. Are there call buttons in the bathrooms and the main areas of the apartment or room(s)?

*Meals*

1. How are special dietary needs met?
2. Do you have assigned seating in the dining room? If so, how are the table companions selected?
3. Are traditional holiday meals observed for our religion?
4. Are residents allowed to take food from the dining area to their apartment or room?
5. What is your policy regarding gratuities?
6. What if my parent wants to have a guest at a meal?
7. What if we want to have a special family celebration?

Questions to ask when hiring a person to come into your home to provide care:

1. How long has your company been in business?
2. Is the agency certified in Medicaid, Medicare, and the Joint Commission on Accreditation of Health Care Organizations, and state licensing boards?
3. Are your workers bonded and insured?
4. What are the charges? Is it an hourly rate or a day rate? Is there overtime pay past a certain amount of hours?
5. What are the company's financial procedures?
6. Does the agency train its own employees?
7. Is there a criminal background check?
8. Can you get information describing services and fees in writing?
9. Does the company have a Licensed Vocational Nurse or RN on staff?
10. Does the staff member I am hiring drive?
11. Does he or she smoke?
12. How will he or she be replaced for days off or vacation time?
13. Am I expected to provide, and pay for, his or her meals?

*Hiring an Independent Caregiver*
Consider the following:

- You are now the employer. Find out what federal, state, and local taxes you are responsible for.
- Will you pay his or her social security tax?
- Which IRS forms need to be filed by you as the employer?

- What will your payment schedule be?
- What if the employee asks for payment earlier than the agreed-to-pay date?
- Are meals included in his/her pay?
- Will you be paying vacation pay or additional holiday pay?
- Have you done a criminal background check on this caregiver?
- Are you satisfied with the references he/she provided?
- Does the caregiver smoke?
- Who will cover for the caregiver during his/her time off?
- Will you allow the caregiver to have visitors in while he/she is caring for your loved one?
- If it is a live-in situation, do you have a separate room and bathroom facilities for the caregiver?
- Do the care receiver have pets? Is the caregiver also responsible for care of the pets?

# CHAPTER 9

# Destination: Your House

*"When you move in with your child, you have to be adaptable. You don't have as much space as you are used to, and you have to shut out some of the things you hear."*

–Anita, 89

## When Your Elderly Parent Moves In

One quarter of all care recipients live with their caregivers, according to a survey by the National Alliance for Caregiving (NAC) and the American Association of Retired Persons, AARP (Pandya, 2005). Once the decision is made to move an elderly relative into the adult child's home, considerations and adjustments need to be made in the family's lifestyle.

Just 20% of parents would choose to move in with their kids, while 63% of adult children say they would have their healthy parents live with them, according to Generations Survey: Parent Child Relationships, a report by Mark Clements Research in 2004.

Several pages of this chapter are dedicated to tactics on keeping the entire family stress free. The sandwich generation is defined, and a new dimension of this family care paradigm, the double-tiered sandwich generation, is introduced.

Prior to a parent's moving in, assessments need to be made regarding the strengths and weaknesses of the rest of the caregiver's family. In the following pages, care receivers who have moved in with their children, discuss why moving in sometimes means falling out. Independence and loss of freedom by the care receiver are also reviewed. For the most part, the elders who are moving in want to continue to have a feeling of self-worth, and to look forward to contributing to their new household in some way. They want to have a feeling of involvement in their child's home, and to continue to "parent" and "grandparent." In some cases, these efforts are welcomed, in others boundaries are breached and authority is questioned.

In this chapter, the new living arrangement is also viewed from the other perspective—that of the caregiver. Adult children are guided through the paces of asking for help and being conscientious about not shouldering the burden of care alone.

Both care receiver and caregiver should be ready for some alterations in the dynamics of their current family relationships. Each individual who takes on the role of primary care provider needs to recognize that once an elderly parent moves in, there will be a shift in who gets the majority of the caregiver's attention.

> *"I always said I would never live with my children. When you are younger, you always want to be independent. Maybe I didn't want to move in with them because I didn't have such a great relationship with my own mother."*
>
> *Anita believes that the aging parent cannot be impervious toward change, and must be accepting of the adult child's lifestyle. "When parents move in with their children ... they have to understand that their children have problems, too. I certainly never want to be a burden to them."*

**—Anita, 89, who has lived with her daughter and son-in-law for 6 years**

### The Entourage of Care

*"Who are all these people?"*    Prepare yourself for a parade of health care professionals who will come and go through your front door to serve your ailing relative's needs. The caregiver and his or her family should be ready for the entourage of care to arrive. The army of helpers could include physical and occupational therapists, visiting nurses, physicians, home health aides, hospice workers, volunteers, and direct medical-equipment delivery people.

### Grab Bars Are Not a Snack

*Home Health and Adaptive Equipment*    The delivery trucks are lined up in the driveway as you make room for the direct medical equipment (DME). Although the devices and equipment needs are individualized for every patient, here is a sampling of what supplies may be needed at your house:

Wheelchair
Hoyer lift
Commode
Elevated toilet seat
Shower chair
Respirator
Grab bars
Oxygen tank
Hospital bed
Walker
Crutches
Pacemaker check kit
Cane
Incontinence products

Assess the space and accessibility in your home for this equipment, including the width of doorways. Caregivers should anticipate that physical changes to their homes might be necessary to make the home more adaptable to the elderly relative. Modifications to the family's bathrooms, entrances and doorways are always a possibility. Check out information about securing a home loan in the event you need modifications such as ramps and larger doorways. Consult your personal banker for loan information.

> When Anita (who was introduced earlier in the chapter) moved into the townhouse with its three levels, she anticipated that walking up and down the stairs to her bedroom could become a problem as her knees become weaker. As a result of her forward thinking, Anita had an electric stair-climbing chair installed between the ground level and living room level of her home. "I only use it if me knees are giving me any trouble."

Using financial strategies and good common sense are a must when considering home renovations and budgeting to meet the financial demands of having another person in the home. Securing a home-equity loan for renovation is one option. The loan can be a good way to pay for repairs. However, since it is secured by your house and property, you could lose your home if you cannot meet the terms of the loan. Make sure you can afford to make the monthly payments.

When investigating loan programs, deal only with reputable lenders. Scam artists prey on the elderly and the uninformed who are looking for ways to build up equity for home renovations.

*Another Mouth to Feed—Looking for Financial Help*

In a 2000 study by the American Society on Aging, respondents who were caregivers reported helping with expenses for 2 to 6 years for a total of an average of $19,525 in out-of-pocket expenses. An interesting and innovative way to bring more money into your household for food and care is to get a reverse mortgage on your home. A reverse mortgage is a loan against your home that requires no repayment of the loan for as long as you live there. To qualify for a reverse mortgage you must:

- Own your own home, and all owners listed on the mortgage must be at least 62 years old. If you are over 62 and moving an elderly parent in with you, their age is not a problem.
- Your home must be your "principal residence." That is, you must live in it more than 6 months of the year.
- For the federally insured "Home Equity Conversion Mortgage (HECM), your home must be a single-family property, a two- to four-unit building, or a federally approved condominium or planned unit development (PUC). Cooperatives and most mobile homes are not eligible. Some "manufactured" homes do qualify if they are built on a permanent foundation and classed and taxed as real estate.
- If you have existing debt against your home, you must pay it off before getting a reverse mortgage, or use an immediate cash advance from the reverse mortgage to pay it off.

Additional information and answers to frequently asked questions about reverse mortgages and home equity loans for renovation are available from the American Association of Retired Persons' (AARP) website, www. aarp.org/revmort/, or the AARP Home Equity Conversion Information Center (202-434-6044). For information from the National Center for Home Equity Conversion (NCHEC), write to them at 7373 147th St., Room 115, Apple Valley MN 55124.

Some cities have interest-free loan programs to finance home repairs for low-income residents. Many non-profit groups, such as Habitat for Humanity, offer home rehabilitation services for the elderly or for families without adequate financial resources. Other resourceful ways to raise cash for home improvements are: borrowing against your life insurance policy or annuity; a low-interest-rate credit card; federal home improvement loans; or state veterans loans. To qualify for a veteran's loan, you must have completed at least 90 days of active military duty.

Having an elderly parent move in can have its financial rewards as well. Earlier in this chapter, you met Anita, who lives with her daughter and son-in law. Anita's move into the town home with her daughter made it financially feasible for both parties to move to a larger home. She says, "I said, 'Listen, I am going to pay rent wherever I go.' Now I help them with the mortgage."

Anita is just one of many care receivers whose move in with the children meant combining two households into a new, larger location. There are many benefits that are beyond financial when moving aging parents in their children's home. The blending of two households can be a benefit for both care receiver and care provider. Anita is an integral part of running the house. "I help with Simon [the dog], and accept packages. I am less of a burden now [living with my daughter], than I was when I lived alone. I was being rushed off to the hospital all the time when I lived alone."

Getting grandparents and grandchildren under the same roof, in many cases, creates a special bonding experience that may not have been present before the entry of the elder. In the case of Edward, a feisty 75-year-old Irishman who is a semi-retired civil engineer, it was his grandparenting initiative that made him move across the country.

A native of Port Chester, New York, Edward lived most of his life on the east coast. In 2004, he moved to Chicago to be closer to his son and to contribute to the positive upbringing of his three grandchildren. Prior to his move, he had mentored his 8-year-old granddaughter in New York on everything she could possibly learn about carpentry and architecture. He took her on many field trips to various construction sites. Although Edward didn't like to leave his granddaughter in New York, he remained optimistic about his move to Chicago. "I've done all I can, but there are three kids [his grandchildren in Chicago] out here who need some parenting and grandparenting. I try to stay out of it, but once in a while, it overcomes me."

### Does the Sandwich Generation Live at Your House?

Sixteen million adults, representing half of all baby boomers ages 45–55, are part of the "sandwich generation." In simple terms, this includes adult children taking care of aging parents while caring for their own children, or who have children living at home while assuming elder care responsibilities. Many Americans in this age group have aging relatives living with them, as well as children under 21. My husband has his own take on where he and I fit within the sandwich generation. We don't have kids, but we were the primary caregivers for my parents. He believes we are the "open-faced" sandwich generation.

### The New Double-Tiered Sandwich Generation

Now that Americans are living longer, another layer of the sandwich generation, the "Double-Tiered Sandwich Generation," has evolved over the last 10 to 20 years. It consists of adult children who are grandparents themselves and are taking care of their own aging parents. Conflict and stress are evident when the adult child resents time spent with an aging parent, and feels that more time could be spent with the grandchildren. These younger grandparents usually are 55–75 years old, with parents who are in their 80s or 90s. They are probably living on a fixed income and helping to shoulder the additional financial burden of the elder relatives.

*What about the Kids?*    Adolescents are one of the elements that add spice to the sandwich (generation). Recognize that once your elderly parent moves in, there may be a power struggle for attention between your child and your parent. Having teenagers living at home adds yet another dimension to possible tension and stress regarding their own mom or dad's attention level.

Help your children understand why your elderly relative's moods may change. Explain to them what happens when their grandfather is in pain. Include your children in the care plan. Give them a chore to help Grandma. Help your child remember new boundaries that are in place regarding noise, privacy, and space. Spend as much time with your kids during this period as possible. Ask for help. If parents of other kids offer to help, take them up on the offer.

### Oh, Brother—Don't Forget Your Siblings

Look to your brothers and sisters for help. Family bonds often become strained when it comes to care management for Mom or Dad. Include everybody. Figure out the strengths and talents of each brother or sister and use those talents. Work as a team. Let past sibling rivalries and resentments stay in the past. Listen to each other. Respect each other's opinions. Include the in-laws. They often want to help. Some relatives just need to be asked. (Read more about siblings working as a team in Chapter 11.)

No two families are alike. Counselors who have worked with families whose loved ones have Alzheimer's disease have put a new spin on the "seen one, seen them all" phrase. They say, "When you've met one Alzheimer's family, you've met *one* Alzheimer's family.

### Living on the Edge

*Living Closer, Not Moving In*    One way Edward, our New York to Chicago transplant "stayed out" of his own son's parenting arena was to have his own apartment just down the street from his son and family. Divorced from his first wife and a widower by his second, Edwards's decision to move was solely his own. He spends the majority of his days at his son's house.

*Jimmy, 85, and his wife, Mabel, 82, left their 30-acre farm in rural Maryland and moved to a two-bedroom condominium in Chicago at the insistence of his stepdaughter, Bobbi. They moved into the same condominium complex where Bobbi lives. Their daughter had become aware that the farm, with its three buildings to maintain, had become too much for her parents to handle. Bobbi was also worried that their rural location would leave them isolated during the next snowy Maryland winter.*

*When you talk with Jimmy, you hear reluctance and acceptance in his voice about the transition and his new surroundings. "Well, there are physical aspects of a farm that age cannot overcome. A farm in Maryland, weather wise, is unsuitable for older people who can't get immediate attention. You can be on a farm, slip, and fall down. You don't have the strength to get up. You don't have the visitors that you would have if you were living in the spot where younger people were constantly in contact with you. So, if I fell down at 8 o'clock in the morning, there are 200 pounds of me that my wife couldn't pick up. It might be too slippery for her to go a quarter of a mile to get some help. There may be no other way. The phone could be down."*

*The scenario regarding a potential accident or illness on the farm was enough to prompt Jimmy and Mabel to move. "It was necessary to make those decisions and the opportunity came along. I thought about the proposition that Bobbi knew about, and we just acted suddenly and have tried to capitalize on that. Even if I did go out and slip and fall now at 8 o'clock in the morning, before 8:15 somebody would have decided I wasn't a drunk lying there. Someone would offer some type of help here in the city. You just couldn't expect help like that in a community like a farm area in Maryland. There's not the number of people there to call upon, much less depend upon. I couldn't expect you as a neighbor to come looking for us every hour or so to see if I was all right or even call me on the phone. You have the same things to do for those who are near and dear to you in your own family."*

## Moving In—Less Space, Less Freedom

For the aging parent who is moving into an adult child's home, the transition doesn't come without compromise and some loss of independence. The senior who once had an entire house to move around in may now be relegated to a bedroom and shared bath. "When I first moved in, my independence was comprised in certain ways," Anita said, in talking about her move. "My daughter was watching me all the time, saying, 'Are you doing too much?' I feel more confident now. It takes time."

Jimmy also felt that his independence had been reduced as a result of his move. "I lost a lot of freedom as far as my own particular activity was concerned. I can't just go to the bank or go shopping for small things that probably never meant anything to anybody. For instance, I lost a pocketknife, which was the last one I had. And it hasn't been replaced yet. Nobody sees any need, any need with a capital 'N', for me to have another. But, it's something I've had all my life and used to use on little things.

" I've got a key ring on here now. With my knife, I'd pry it open, put the two rings together and be through with it in 3 minutes. Now, it takes me sometimes 2025 minutes to try to get that key ring open, because I have nothing small like that. I don't want to use these stainless steel knives because they end up bending. They're not good. That's the kind of freedom I miss."

## The Ties that Bind

*Making Your Family Members Stress Free*   A critical first step to take before the move-in takes place is to open the lines of communication among you, your aging parent, and the rest of the family. Try to be proactive about conflict and emotional situations that could arise. For Anita, that meant a mother-to-daughter talk early on. "We talked about it. And we decided that if we had anything on our minds, we would sit down and discuss it." Anita feels that the move has brought her daughter closer emotionally. She also believes that the efforts for all to live in harmony can't be one-sided. "My daughter is not too easy to get along with. Sometimes she can be flippant and caustic. The parent has to learn to give a little bit, too. It's a trade off. I understand her, and she tells me, 'Mother, that's the way I am.'"

Your home may start to feel a little crowded. Maybe your kids, or you and your spouse have to give up a bathroom. Discuss who's giving up their room. Decisions need to be made about family laundry, extra supplies, family meals, special diets, and privacy.

One more thought about space. If you don't have a spare bedroom on the first floor, the family dining room often is a great spot to convert for an aging parent. It is usually on the first floor, is spacious, and has a wide doorway. Some even have multiple doorways. In the days of yesteryear, or at least in the 1950s, my ailing great-grandmother moved into her dining room, hospital bed and all, where she "held court" until her dying day.

*Action Steps to Keep Harmony in the Home*

- Have a family meeting *before* your loved one moves in.
- Make a plan regarding who will let the medical personnel in and out.
- Decide which areas of the home are off limits to the new help.
- If you have children living in the home, set aside personal time with them.
- Plan some family activities that don't revolve around your elderly parent.
- Make sure that your family pets know about some of the new boundaries.
- Have your family plan include times when loud music should be avoided, or children's friends should not come over.
- Try to keep the family's current schedule for activities intact.
- Check out respite programs for your elderly loved one when the time comes for a family vacation.

*Family Fallout That Turns to Elder Abuse*

Several entries in this book address elder abuse and neglect. The topic is covered more extensively in Chapter 12. But it is focused on here because a frail individual can become extremely vulnerable when moving into a family member's home. The elderly individual could become exposed to potential volatile situations that can result in abuse or neglect. Too often, a caregiver can reach a breaking point with the result that the elder suffers the consequences.

An arresting fact revealed in the Department of Health & Human Services Administration on Aging's 1998 National Elder Abuse Incidence Study shows that among known perpetrators of abuse and neglect, the perpetrator was a family member in 90% of cases. Two-thirds of them were adult children or spouses.

Every effort has to be made to not let any situation get out of hand where abuse, neglect, or exploitation can happen. If there are other family members living in the home who have a history of violence or exploitation, alternate arrangements should be made for the elderly loved one.

Reporting incidents of abuse is critical. Often the frail, vulnerable victims of abuse are too humiliated to do self-reporting. In many instances, the elderly relative doesn't want to expose an abusive son or daughter.

National Center on Elder Abuse
1201 Fifteenth Street NW, Suite 350
Washington, DC 20005-2842
(202) 898-2586
www.elderabusecenter.org

In addition to the national Center on Elder Abuse listed previously, the local social service agencies, police departments and hospitals will get involved in abuse cases when reported. The following table includes toll free numbers for reporting elder abuse out of state. If the number listed is for in-state calls only, call the Eldercare Locator at 800-677-1116.

### Don't Go It Alone—Ask for Help

Having your elderly loved one move in may be the result of an illness or because they can no longer can physically take care of themselves. As the caregiver, don't hesitate to bring in outside help.

Hiring a home aide doesn't have to be financially out of reach. Many agencies have sliding scale payment programs, depending on a person's income. Some organizations offer volunteers who can help with your caregiving chores.

Assess how much help you will need. Do you need someone to come in for a couple of hours, so that you can run some errands? Does your loved one need 24-hour care and help with grooming, incontinence or transferring?

### Bringing in the Hired Hands

*Do You Need Home Care Or Health Care?*    *Home Care* services are those that are custodial, such as cleaning, laundry, escorts, sitters, bathing, brushing teeth, toileting, and dressing.

*Health Care* services include physical therapy, speech, catheterization, respite care, medication monitoring, wound care, and occupational therapy.

There are two methods for employing paid caregivers in your home.

1. An individual hired through an agency. These individuals are usually licensed and bonded, and the agency can get a replacement if your caregiver is sick or late. The cost is much higher for agency help, but there are benefits.
2. An independent caregiver. You take your chances when you hire someone independently. Who will replace them for time off? What if they don't show up? Has there been a background check? The daily/weekly charge is much less than hiring through an agency.

There are many questions to ask when hiring a home care agency or overseeing a private-duty aide. (Some of these questions are similar to those in Chapter 6, but are covered here from a different perspective. Cross-reference the questions in Chapter 6).

*Action Steps for Hiring*

Have a written agreement about pay schedule, severance pay, advance pay, and who will administer the checks.

- Does the individual smoke?
- Are your household pets a problem?
- Will he have a replacement for days off?
- Will you allow the aide to have visitors?
- Who is responsible for personal phone calls made by the aide?
- Make a plan about the aide's meals.
- Talk to your accountant about paid caregivers and taxes.
- Talk to your insurance agent about coverage in case the caregiver is injured in your home.

Welcoming an aging loved one into your home comes with an obvious, yet unspoken question: How long will the visit last? The answer can't be given in black and white or definitive terms. The ailing relative will stay until death? Until nursing home placement becomes necessary? Until he or she is well enough to go out independently into the world again?

To ensure that the ties that bind a family together don't become frayed because of the elderly relative who has moved in, communication is key. Elderly people want the freedom to continue to live lives that are familiar and comfortable. Primary caregivers must monitor their own sensory overload levels. With enough advance planning, open discussion, and respect for each family member's needs, the multigenerational family can thrive together under one roof.

Toll Free Hotlines (last updated August 17, 2005)

| State | Domestic Elder Abuse | Institutional Elder Abuse | Accessibility | Comments |
|---|---|---|---|---|
| Alabama | 800-458-7214 | | In-state only | Accepts referrals 18+ |
| Alaska | 800-478-9996 907-269-3666 | 800-730-6393 907-334-4483 | In-state only Nationwide | |
| Arizona | 877-767-2385 | 877-767-2385 | Nationwide | TDD 877-815-8390 |
| Arkansas | 800-332-4443 | 800-582-4887 | Nationwide | In-state hotline can be called from out of state at 800-482-8049 Accepts referrals 18+ |
| California | 888-436-3600 | 800-231-4024 | In-state only | Adult Protective Services County Contact List |
| Colorado | 800-773-1366 | 800-773-1366 800-886-7689 | In-state only | Accepts referrals 18+ |
| Connecticut | 888-385-4225 | 860-424-5241 | In-state only | Domestic Elder Abuse, serves age 60 or older. LTC facilities, serve those 18 years and older. Toll free # for Domestic Elder Abuse during business hours. After hours, CT residents call Info line at 211. |
| Delaware | 800-223-9074 | 800-223-9074 | Nationwide | Accepts referrals for 18+ |
| D.C. | 202-541-3950 | 202-434-2140 | | Accepts referrals 18+ |
| Florida | 800-962-2873 | 800-962-2873 | Nationwide | |
| Georgia | 888-774-0152 404-657-5250 | 800-878-6442 404-657-5728 | Nationwide Metro Atlanta | 8am–5pm; M-F |
| Guam | 671-475-0268 | 671-475-0268 | | On weekends, holidays & between the hours 5p.m.–8 a.m. On weekdays, call 671-646-4455 |

| State | | | | |
|---|---|---|---|---|
| Hawaii | 808-832-5115<br>808-243-5151<br>808-241-3432<br>808-933-8820<br>808-327-6280 | Same | Oahu<br>Maui<br>Kauai<br>EastHawaii<br>West Hawaii | |
| Idaho | 877-471-2777<br>208-334-3833 | 877-471-2777<br>208-364-1899 | Nationwide<br>In state only | M–F 8 a.m.–5 p.m. |
| Illinois | 217-524-6911<br>800-252-8966 | 217-785-0321<br>800-252-4343 | Nationwide<br>In-state only | After hours, report domestic abuse at 800-279-0400 or Elder Care Locator 800-677-1116 |
| Indiana | 800-992-6978 | 800-992-6978 | In-state only<br>Out of state, call 800-545-7763, ext. 20135 | Accepts referrals 18+ |
| Iowa | 800-362-2178 | 877-686-0027 | Nationwide 800#<br>In-state only | Accepts referrals 18+ |
| Kansas | 800-922-5330<br>785-296-0044 | 800-842-0078 | In-state only<br>Out of state | Long-Term Care Ombudsman: 877-662-8362 (In-state only) or 785-296-3017 (Out of state) Mental Health and Developmental Disabilities: 800-221-7923 |
| Kentucky | *800-752-6200 | *800-752-6200<br>**800-372-2991 | In-state only | *Abuse Hotline<br>#**LTC Ombudsman |

(Continued)

Toll Free Hotlines (last updated August 17, 2005)

| State | Domestic Elder Abuse | Institutional Elder Abuse | Accessibility | Comments |
|---|---|---|---|---|
| Louisiana | 800-259-4990 | 800-259-4990 | In-state only | |
| Maine | 800-624-8404 | 800-624-8404 | Nationwide | Accepts referrals 18+ |
| Maryland | 800-917-7383<br>800-677-1116 | 800-917-7383<br>877-402-8220 | In-state only<br>Nationwide | |
| Massachusetts | 800-922-2275 | 800-462-5540 | In-state only | |
| Michigan | 800-996-6228 | 800-882-6006 | In-state only | |
| Minnesota | 800-333-2433 | 800-333-2433 | Nationwide | Referral to Senior LINKAGE LINE and county service |
| Mississippi | 800-222-8000 | 800-227-7308 | Domestic:<br>In-state only | Institutional - Nationwide |
| Missouri | 800-392-0210 | 800-392-0210 | Nationwide | Accepts referrals 18+ |
| Montana | 800-551-3191<br>406-444-4077 | None available | In-state only<br>Nationwide | |
| Nebraska | 800-652-1999 | 800-652-1999 | In-state only | Accepts referrals 18+ with functional or mental impairments |
| Nevada | 800-992-5757 | 800-992-5757 | In-state only | Reno area:<br>702-784-8090 |
| New Hampshire | 800-949-0470<br>603-271-4386 | 800-442-5640<br>603-271-4396 | In-state only<br>Out of state | |
| New Jersey | 800-792-8820<br>609-943-3473 | 800-792-8820<br>609-943-3473 | In-state only<br>Nationwide | |

| State | | | | |
|---|---|---|---|---|
| New Mexico | 800-797-3260<br>505-841-6100 | 800-797-3260<br>505-841-6100 | In-state only<br>Albuquerque & Out-of-state | |
| New York | *800-342-9871 | Nursing Home Complaint<br>888-201-4563<br>Adult Care Home Complaint<br>866-893-6772 | Nationwide<br>In-state only | *For in-state referrals during business hrs. choose "OPTION 6" Local county Depts. of Social Services offices |
| North Carolina | 800-662-7030 | 800-662-7030 | In-state only | |
| North Dakota | 800-451-8693 | 800-451-8693 | Nationwide | |
| Ohio | 866-635-3748<br>800-677-1116 | 800-282-1206<br>800-677-1116 | Nationwide<br>Out-of-state | |
| Oklahoma | 800-522-3511 | 800-522-3511 | In-state only | 24 hours, 7 days |
| Oregon | 800-232-3020 | 800-232-3020 | In-state only | Mental health & Developmental disabilites - 866-406-4287 |
| Pennsylvania | 800-490-8505 | 800-254-5164 | Nationwide | |
| Puerto Rico | 787-725-9788<br>787-721-8225 | | | |
| Rhode Island | 401-462-0550<br>401-462-0545 (fax) | 401-785-3340<br>401-785-3391 (fax) | In-state only | Accepts referrals for elders 60+ M–F 8:30 a.m.–4 p.m. |

*(Continued)*

Toll Free Hotlines (last updated August 17, 2005)

| State | Domestic Elder Abuse | Institutional Elder Abuse | Accessibility | Comments |
|---|---|---|---|---|
| South Carolina | None Available | None Available | | Suspected abuse or neglect: contact local Adult Protective Services/DSS office. DSS Online Directory. Report nursing home abuse: local Long Term Care Ombudsman Office/Area Agency on Aging AAA Online Directory |
| South Dakota | 605-773-3656 | 605-773-3656 | | M-F 8 a.m.–5 p.m. |
| Tennessee | 888-277-8366 | 888-277-8366 | Nationwide | Ages 18+ who are impaired |
| Texas | 800-252-5400 512-834-3784 | 800-458-9858 512-834-3784 | Nationwide Out of state | |
| Utah | 801-264-7669 800-371-7897 | 801-264-7669 800-371-7897 | Nationwide In-state only | M–F, 8:00a.m.– 5:00p.m. |
| Vermont | 800-564-1612 | 800-564-1612 | In-state only | |
| Virgin Islands | None available | None available | | |
| Virginia | 888-832-3858 804-371-0896 | 888-832-3858 804-371-0896 | In-state only Out of state | Hotline available 24 hours, 7 days a week Online www.seniornavigator .com |
| Washington | 866-363-4276 | 800-562-6078 | Nationwide | Info. 800-422-3263 APS Regional intake numbers |
| West Virginia | 800-352-6513 | 800-352-6513 | In-state only | |
| Wisconsin | 608-266-2536 | 800-815-0015 608-246-7013 800-677-1116 | 800#s: In-state only Out of state | Guardianship: 800-488-2596 or 608-224-0660 Consumer Protection: 800-422-7128 |
| Wyoming | 800-457-3659 307-777-6137 | 307-777-7123 | In-state only | Referrals to local agency - State LTC Ombudsman 307-322-5553 |

# CHAPTER 10

# A Million Miles Away:
# Receiving Care from a Distance

*We haven't quite reached that point that we expect help all the time. But our children are all out of town. One is living in California, one in Phoenix, and one in Chicago. They're wonderful to offer help if we need it. And they'll come home occasionally just to visit. But, again, we just don't want to be real dependent. I think down the road, at our age, and with our health, that we're not going to be independent and, yeah, I am wondering about exactly how we're going to handle it.*

—Fred (pseudonym), 83

For adult children who are unable to be physically present during their parents' journey through frailty and illness, the stress factor is very high. They worry about whether the parents are getting the right medication, getting enough food, are in a secure location, and whether their cognitive functioning is declining.

Gone are the days of generations growing up, marrying, and raising new families in the same old neighborhood. As the baby boomer generation and their children become more global, families become separated by distance. It is our elders who, more often than not, are the ones who "stay put."

An estimated 7 million to 10 million adult children are caring for their parents by long distance. This chapter answers many questions for those caregivers, and provides referral sources for contacting geriatric-care managers. Sometimes called, "the other daughter," professional care managers can be a blessing if you live away from your aging parent.

As mentioned above, millions of Americans provide services for an older adult who lives at least 1 hour away, according to a survey cosponsored by The National Council on the Aging (NCOA) and The Pew Charitable Trusts. The number of long-distance caregivers is expected to double over the next 15 years as the baby boomers and their parents age, according to the NCOA statistics.

The same NCOA survey provides a snapshot of the average care recipient receiving long-distance help as 78 years old; 64% are women. The care recipient was typically a relative of the caregiver: 53% were parents or stepparents, 11% were grandparents, 10% were adult children, and 16% were other relatives.

On average, the care receivers lived 304 miles away from the care providers. Those who managed the care spent an average of 4 hours traveling to reach the person who needed help. Older boomers (age 43 to 51) are more likely than younger boomers and the population in general to provide long-distance care.

### Care Management Through the Internet

*Guess Who's on Line?*   Many seniors have become acquainted with the Internet to strengthen the ties that bind, and to communicate with loved ones. According to a source for Nielsen/Net Ratings (2003), senior citizens are the fastest growing group of Internet users. In a 2002 survey conducted by SeniorNet of 2,084 (2002) people in the United States age 50 and older, 94% of seniors use the 'Net to communicate with friends and family. While on-line communication with relatives is the elders' first priority, the second most popular search for seniors on the Web is to check on news and events.

One technology company has even invented a cyber-nanny that is run by microchips and sensors for the dependent elderly person. The device can detect whether the ailing person has fallen or is non-responsive, and it can summon help. This high-tech companion can even sense if a burner on the stove has been left on, and can switch lights on and off from another room. Don't look for this aide in your local discount stores anytime soon. This device is in the prototype phase, and is several years away from distribution.

Home security companies such as ADT have devised systems for the elderly market that are also activated by motion in the home. The ADT QuietCare Plus system uses small wireless motion detectors placed in strategic locations throughout the home such as the master bath, bedroom, kitchen and medication area. Each sensor transmits information about the senior's daily living activities 24 hours a day, 7 days a week. Caregivers and family members can receive the information through telephone calls, cell phone text messaging and e-mail.

## Covering the Bases

It is important that long-distance caregivers do plenty of work up front to make their loved ones' environment safe. Perhaps this is the time to give your parents' trustworthy neighbor a set of keys. There are a number of emergency response systems on the market and home care agencies that can aid in a dependent person's safety. Another concern for long-distance caregivers is keeping harmony with siblings and other caregivers who are located near parents and can observe them full time. Sometimes those who come from a distance have a completely different perspective on how things at a parent's home should be handled.

Family dynamics in respect to relationships can also reveal "prodigal" sons and daughters, who are those children who aren't involved in the caregiving process at all, but who the parent misses and cherishes so much. When a family member must be cared for long distance, it is not the time for siblings to bring up past histories or rivalries. Team effort is critical.

## Semipermanent Visits

When adult children live miles apart in different states, working out visits with the parents sometimes takes creativity. Some siblings have worked out a rotation schedule where the parent spends several months at each child's home. The advantage of this arrangement is having grandparents spend extended quality time with grandchildren. Having the aging parent come for an extended visit allows the adult child to continue his or her usual routine at home.

This kind of rotation schedule doesn't work for everyone. For an elderly parent who may have dementia or limited mobility, traveling is difficult. In addition, with any form of Alzheimer's disease, it could be harmful to take the older adult out of his or her own familiar environment.

## Long Distance Care: A Two-Way Street

When aging relatives live out of state and need care, either they can travel to the adult child; or a younger relative, such as a niece or nephew, can set up camp at the ailing elder's home. Moving the dependent elderly individual away on a permanent basis from what is familiar can cause anxiety about making new friends, finding a new church, and establishing new relationships with doctors. You will need some assurance that their medical coverage is transferable, and that there is easy access to medical professionals in the new area.

In the majority of cases, however, it is the younger, more able family member who picks up and either moves to the home of the dependent elder, or visits frequently enough to manage the elder's care.

> I wish we had family closer. Our children all live in different states. They are wonderful about trying to come home, and they do, and have, every time we've needed them. I can't expect them to do that just on a whim. They have a lot of things going on in their lives that sometimes it just can't be convenient for them. So that bothers me. We have a lot of friends who have children who live in town, and we see how wonderful that is. Well, as I say, they have said that if we ever need them they will come.
>
> But, no, I don't expect my children to move. I feel like my mother. I moved away and left my parents, and they never complained. I was able, fortunately, to come home when my mother was real ill and also my father, but that doesn't always happen. But the timing was so I could, and I had a husband that understood.
>
> [Our children] really try to call often and find out what's going on and they care a lot. We're very fortunate. They really do care, but it's not like having them live here. But I would never, never imply that I want them to move here.

—Delores (pseudonym), 82

If the care receiver has no spouse, or that spouse is unable to provide help and there is no family support system locally, the need for long distance relatives to intervene is that much greater. Doing so, however, can be very costly both emotionally and financially.

### One Daughter's Road Trip

The following is one adult daughter's account of her long-distance travels in 2004 and 2005. Over 10 months, Marian traveled by car three different times, and once by airplane, from her home in Thousand Oaks, California to Shreveport, Louisiana—1,663.6 miles *one way*—to care for her ailing 84 year-old mother, Johanna. In 2005, she spent 3 months in Shreveport as her mother transitioned from an independent apartment through an extended hospital stay and finally into a nursing home.

The youngest of five children, Marian has four siblings located in Shreveport, Chicago, Dallas, and Virginia. Although her oldest brother makes the trip from Dallas to Shreveport at least once and sometimes twice a month, it is Marian who has logged in the most miles and extended stays.

Marian's first journey to Shreveport in 2004 to "officially" tend to her mother was combined with some family vacation and a stop in Chicago for a family reunion. Her subsequent trips to Shreveport were made out of necessity to address immediate care problems regarding her mother.

> I drove with my son, Greg, 22, and daughter, Sarah, 19, from Thousand Oaks to Las Vegas, Nevada, and spent 3 days there with them. Greg then flew back to college and Sarah drove on with me to Chicago. After four days in Chicago, we picked up a friend who had flown in from Malibu to drive the rest of the trip with me. We headed on down to Shreveport, a 15-hour drive. We spent 5 days in Shreveport, and had a little family reunion of sorts with all my siblings. Then we drove back by way of Texas and Arizona. I put about 3,600 miles on my car during this trip. The time frame of that trip was from the end of July 2004 until mid August 2004.
>
> My next car trip to Shreveport happened as a result of my mom's demon cat attacking her. Mom wound up in the emergency room, ripped apart, bitten, and needing stitches. The cat was destroyed by animal services, and my mother went into a depressive tailspin after that. So I hopped into my car again. It was two 12-hour days and about a 6-hour day to drive there, and 1,700-plus miles on my car.
>
> I stayed with my mom in her apartment for 3 weeks, until the end of September. She was quite depressed while healing from the cat attack. She did not want to discuss getting another cat, saying "maybe later." Since I still had my job at the hospital (I was a "per diem" employee and had an open, nebulous schedule), I did need to get back home after a 3-week absence, to work for about 10 days at my job. So I drove from Shreveport to Dallas and left my car with my sister-in-law. Flew home from Dallas, worked the 10 days, flew back to Dallas and then spent the night with another sister-in-law. Since I now had my car again, I then pushed on back to Shreveport.
>
> By now, my mom said she was ready to get another cat. I had been praying that God would lead me to just the right animal for her, since that last demon cat had been such a disaster—he had bitten and scratched her numerous times and she would hide it like an abused spouse hides the beatings from a husband or wife. I was led to an ad in the paper, to a cat that was sweet, lovable, and calm. The cat became "Elsie" and Mom was thrilled. Elsie took right to her and was the perfect "lap cat" companion my mom needed. I stayed another week, and then drove back to California.

In March of 2005, Marian's road trips began again when her mother was hospitalized in Shreveport with complications from a mild heart attack. This time, all of the adult children gathered at their mother's bedside because the prognosis looked bleak. Johanna's extended stay at the hospital included therapy and tests for dementia.

After considering many outcomes upon discharge from the hospital, Johanna, along with her children, decided that a nursing home would be the place to live. During her 6-week hospitalization, Marian stayed in her mother's apartment, and then stayed on another 4 weeks to get her mother settled in the nursing home.

Marian's long drive back to Thousand Oaks wasn't without incident. When she broke a crown off a tooth, she drove straight to her brother's periodontal office in Dallas. "That was the last straw," she says. "He ended up doing a 'crown-lengthening procedure' and I drove back across the country having to chew on one side, with stitches and discomfort on the other side."

Shortly after she returned home, a letter, written in pencil, arrived from her mother. It read, "Dear Mare. Is your mouth without pain at least? I'm so sorry that happened to you. My new room is just like the one I had—but backwards. I go to the dining room 3 times a day. Treatment is royal here. Let me know how you, your dear husband, Michael, and 'Elsie' are. Love, Mom"

After her total 3-month stay in Shreveport, Marian was back in California. Her nerves were frayed, and she could feel depression rearing its ugly head. Her caregiving journey has been a bumpy road. Elsie, the cat, remained in Shreveport with a foster family.

*Caregiving across Oceans and Continents*

Long-distance caregiving takes on a whole new meaning when the care management dyad extends between two countries. Looking out for relatives from outside the country where you live presents a host of practical and logistical problems. The travel expenses, anxiety of not getting back to a loved one before it's too late, and not knowing the true nature of your loved one's condition are compounded when you are overseas.

Samir, 77, and his wife, Fatima, 72 (not their real names), are medical professionals whose practices are in their native Tehran, the capital of Iran. Their three adult children have taken up permanent residency in the United States.

For 3 months out of the year, Samir and Fatima live and work in Iran, more than 8,000 miles away from their children and grandchildren. The rest of the year, they rotate among the homes of their children—two in the Midwest and one in the Rocky Mountains.

Fatima talks about the elderly people in Iran whose adult children have moved to other countries. "They are left behind. Iran families do come back and take care of them. But, sometimes, after the revolution, the older relatives who are left are obliged to go to the nursing homes. When some of the adult children have left the country illegally because of religious persecution or political issues, there is no way for them to come back." In some cases, extended family who still reside in Iran are asked to become care providers.

Fatima also explained that when her mother-in-law became ill in Iran, it was the mother's adult sons—not the daughters-in-law, who took charge. "They knew she would be more comfortable if her blood relatives were providing the care." When the time comes for Samir and Fatima to retire, where will they choose to grow old? "We will retire to the United States to be near our children."

## Getting Your Relative's Affairs in Order

It is never too soon to get copies of your parents' advance directives regarding end-of-life decisions, wills, and financial information. However, a calm and positive discussion needs to take place about privacy issues and your intent in needing this information.

Numbers and information that you should have access to include contact information for their physicians, attorneys, financial planners, and bankers. Find out where your parents bank. Where are the safe-deposit box keys kept?

If your relative is a savvy Internet traveler and possibly keeps all of his or her personal financial information on a computer, you may need to ask for the computer password. It would be an unfortunate turn of events if your loved one leaves specific instructions to be followed upon his death and that all information is logged into a computer that no one can access. Advance planning could be easily lost without the appropriate password. Getting the password while your relative is alive and coherent can be a delicate problem, because some computer users guard this information and don't want their privacy invaded.

## Securing Local Professional Help

If there are no relatives or friends who can be called upon locally for assistance with care, many home care agencies have staff available for various chores and services.

Geriatric care managers have a very strong network across the country. The services geriatric care managers offer run the gamut from conducting home visits, to helping with long-term care facility placement. Information on how to access the National Association of Professional Geriatric Care Managers is located near the end of this chapter.

*Tips on Securing Good Care Management Help*

- Know what they have to offer. Do they specialize in assessments? Are they going to send your case to an outside contractor?
- Get references. Ask for names and phone number of other clients. If they are worth their salt, they will willingly provide this information.
- Assess their style. Their case managers are going to be talking to your loved one about sensitive issues. Make sure they are a good "personality fit."
- Discuss fees. You don't want to be hit with surprises. Do they require a deposit? Who pays—you or your loved one?
- Follow up. Be the "squeaky wheel." If you aren't getting the answers you want to hear, make a change.

For assistance with financial matters and for getting your loved one's bills paid on time, a pool of financial counselors called daily money managers (DMMs) have emerged in the last few years. The DMM is a personal financial assistant who specializes in helping seniors manage their day-to-day personal finances. They can deliver a wide range of services including sorting the mail, paying the bills, delivering bank deposits, and balancing the checkbook, as well as completing insurance forms and tax documents.

As with any professional with whom your family member is sharing confidential information, check credentials and rely on referrals from people you know and trust. Contact your local Area Agency on Aging for referrals, or call 800-677-1116 for your area's agency on aging.

*Action Steps*

- Sit down and have a discussion with the elderly person. The best time to do this is before help is needed. Find out whether there is a plan in place for the future.
- With the dependent elderly individual *included*, hold a family conference about how your family's long-distance caregiving needs are going to be met.
- Together with your family members, weigh and present the options about who, if anyone, will relocate. Will it be your dependent parent? Will it be you or one of your siblings?
- If you have been living away from ailing relatives for a while, get an assessment of how they have been getting along up to this point. Is their home being well cared for? Has their appearance changed? Enlist the help of neighbors.
- Talk to members of your parent's social network, such as church committees, card-playing groups, walking clubs. Ask for their help in

making visits, providing an occasional meal, and contacting you if they see a need for your help.

- Geriatric-case managers have a very supportive network across the country. By calling their national office, you will be able to find out who can help in your relative's local area. Contact the National Association of Professional Geriatric Care Managers, 1604 N. Country Club Road, Tucson, AZ, 85716. 520-881-8008. www.caremanager.org.

The Family Caregiver Alliance distributes a wonderful resource booklet, *New Handbook for Long-Distance Caregivers*. It is free of charge. www.caregiver.org. Hardcopy FCA Publication Order, 180 Montgomery Street Suite 1100 San Francisco, CA, 94104.

Caring for an ailing relative who lives hundreds of miles away brings a challenging new dynamic to the mix. First and foremost, care receivers need to be involved in every decision being made in their behalf. Sensitive privacy issues need to be discussed openly and early on on the care plan. If there are no family members, locally or long distance, who can help, professional care managers should be enlisted. There is help out there for everyone. By doing some research and taking advantage of the resources available to long-distance caregivers, you'll find the distance between you and your loved one shrinking.

CHAPTER **11**

# Circling the Wagons

*I never knew what it was like to have a sister or brother. I was determined when I started to have children not to have only one child. Now, my son and daughter are very close. They talk about everything. When I feel that they are doing too much for me, they say, "Mom, you were always there for us."*

—Anita, 89, an only child

## Adult Children Responding as a Caregiving Team

Teamwork, defined as "each doing a part, but all subordinating personal prominence to the efficiency of the whole," seems like something brothers and sisters could master. Yet, rare is the household that didn't have siblings growing up together who squabbled over toys, attention, and boundaries. It's not surprising that brothers and sisters with elderly parents find themselves at the epicenter of care.

Among family caregivers, adult children are most likely to assume the role of primary caregiver according to a report by The Center on an Aging Society, Georgetown University. In 1999, adult children accounted for 44% of primary family caregivers, the largest proportion of primary caregivers to people age 65 or older. More than 7 million adult children are primary caregivers to their parents.

As the care matrix unfolds, with siblings serving as primary and secondary caregivers for their aging parents, their individual and collective roles are not without conflict. Thrusting brothers and sisters into the endless jobs of homecare assistant, medication monitor, chauffeur, housekeeper, accountant and home security chief, all for the sake of an elderly parent's well-being, can rattle the best of organized teams.

How is a family with siblings of all ages and varied geographic locations to arrange the myriad chores of managing the health and welfare of a frail aging parent? Answer: very carefully, with compassion, understanding, and open communication.

Many families continue to observe rituals and traditions that have always been present in their homes. Keeping siblings to a routine—dinner together at a favorite restaurant; sisters shopping together on a regular basis—will keep the lines of communication open when stressful situations about parental care arise. It had been a tradition in our family that Thanksgiving dinner was cooked and served in my grandmother's home. When her poor health left her incapable of hosting the holiday dinner, her children rallied to the task. My mother, her brothers, and her sister-in-law each made a dish. The turkey was cooked at our house, and transported to my grandmother's house, and the tradition stayed intact. Thanksgiving would always be at Grandma's.

For Anita, (introduced above), the tradition of going out for dinner every Friday night with her children and their spouses is a treat. "We have such a good time together, and we discuss everything—anything that is on our minds!"

## All Siblings Are Not Created Equal

There is usually one adult child who shoulders the majority of the caregiving burden. That child could be the elderly parent's favorite, or the one who handles communication with the parent in the best way. Fifty-three percent of primary caregivers are adult daughters. If she is unmarried and living with the care recipient, she is most likely the child who assumes the role of primary caregiver, according to the report from the Center on an Aging Society (2005).

Don't be surprised if your siblings call upon you because of your particular area of expertise—whatever it may be. If you have special skills in legal counsel, accounting, or health care, your siblings could assume that you will tackle those special tasks for your loved one—whether you choose to or not. If you are usually the "take charge" person in your family, these additional credentials may seal the deal that you will take the lead with many arduous responsibilities. Lustbader and Hooyman (1994) found that, "If the family leader also happens to be a nurse, social worker, physician, or other health professional, siblings usually expect this person to apply these skills to their parents' care."

*The "Prodigal" Ones*

If you haven't experienced this in your own family, you may have heard about it from friends or other extended family. This is the scenario: a son or daughter is acting as the full-time caregiver for an ailing parent, looking after personal care, errands, medication set-up, financial assistance, and so on. Somewhere out there is another adult sibling who doesn't contribute to the care, doesn't show up very often, and is fairly estranged from the whole family caregiving scene. It is this distant child, however, that the elderly parent cherishes. She waits for his phone call or card. When this child does make a rare visit, the parent perks up, and seems to thrive. In other instances, the "prodigal child" doesn't show up until after the parent's death.

Can you sense that there will be resentment on the part of the full-time caregiver in these situations? Absolutely. This family dynamic isn't something you are going to be able to turn around. It probably has a long history. If you find yourself in the role of primary caregiver when a prodigal returns, take advantage of the out-of-towner's visit and give yourself a break. You might say, "As long as you are here with Mom, I'm going to run out for a couple of hours. I'll be back by 5." This opportunity will provide you with some much-needed respite and will take you away from a situation that could become confrontational.

Another task to put into place during the visit from the estranged brother or sister is to conduct the family meeting right then and there while you can include him or her as part of the team. Keep your personal resentment and anger in check. The reaction from your sibling may surprise you.

*"Only" Children—The Team of One*

> *It went through my head many times. Who can I rely on if I have problems? I definitely thought of my [only] son Jim. I always wanted more, but I was only blessed with one. I'm so proud of him.*

> —Charlotte Z. 94

An adult child who has no siblings often feels the need to be "the whole team" when it comes to providing care for an aging parents. For the majority of their lives, it has only been "the three of them" or even the only child and one parent. The caregiving universe is much smaller for this family unit.

Only children may have more feelings of guilt or resentment than their multi-sibling counterparts, because the only child feels they have to "do it all" with little back-up help. Or, there can be guilty feelings or thoughts of abandonment if the adult child wants to live away from the aging parent. In many families, the aging parents will relocate and retire closer to the only child.

Solutions to these feelings of isolation for the only child can be found in enlisting the help of extended family (cousins, nieces, nephews) or community service organizations. Church groups and volunteers can also become part of an extended family and help with some of the caregiving tasks. Hospices also offer volunteers who will visit your loved one and give you a few hours of respite.

Shortly after World War II ended, five young couples moved into a neighborhood called Brighton Park on the southwest side of Chicago. Although all were strangers at move-in time, the new residents became great neighbors and lifelong friends. Over the years, their children played together and became best friends. All of these post-war "baby boomer" children lived with their parents until they married.

An odd coincidence about these five couples is that each couple produced only one child. The five "only-children," most with children of their own now, have remained close over the 6 decades of their lives. "We were like each other's brothers and sisters. We are all still very close today and attend some family functions together," said Lori, 63, one of the five "only" children.

Of the five sets of parents, only two individuals are still alive. One of the men, in his late 80s, continues to live in the original home he bought in Brighton Park over 60 years ago. Charlotte, 94, is the other surviving parent from the Brighton Park group. Until three strokes made it necessary for her to live in a skilled nursing facility, Charlotte lived with her son and daughter-in-law in the small town of Morris, Illinois, about 60 miles south of Chicago. She and her son had both given up their homes in Brighton Park to move to a larger house that could accommodate the blended family. Charlotte's son, Jim, made the decision to move his mother to his new home when the drive to her home became a burden. "I couldn't keep running in [to the city] and continue taking care of two households."

Charlotte loves to reminisce about their happy years with the Brighton Park neighbors and all the children. "All of our kids became each other's brothers and sisters. As long as they could play together, they were all very happy."

### The Out-of-Towners

Adult children who live out of town, away from their ailing parents' day-to-day care, get a swift dose of reality when arriving at the parents home. Perhaps their parent had been healthy and vibrant during a prior visit. If you are the "in-town" care provider, your parent's visible declining health can often spark resentment, guilt, and annoyance on the part of your sibling who has just come home.

As a result of these feelings, the brother or sister who has just arrived on the scene may lash out about how care management has been handled up until this point. *Lustbader and Hooyman (1994)* found that, "Visiting family members often do not consider that they are witnessing the outcome of incremental adaptations rather than irresponsible care." The visiting adult child sees drastic changes; the everyday caregiver may see only slight changes in a parent's health.

Each sibling needs to reassess his or her own role in the caregiving matrix before criticizing the actions of the other siblings. At this point, a family conference with all of the siblings should be convened to sort out how the shortfalls, if any exist, can be corrected.

### Who Has the Time?

Whether siblings are full-time homemakers or corporate CEOs, each has a portion of their lives dedicated to their livelihoods. Conflicts arise with siblings and elderly parents when there are misconceptions about each person's "work" time. For example, there may be resentment from siblings who work full time outside the home about other siblings who work from a home office. Or, for example, a stay-at-home dad may be judged by the other siblings as having more free time to spend tending to the ailing parent than his brothers who are "company men."

The discord over management of caregiving time should be worked out early through a family conference on the care management plan. All brothers and sisters, as well as other relatives who can help shoulder the burden of care, should be included in this meeting.

Angie, 87, lives with her daughter, son in-law, and granddaughter. Her daughter, Pat, and granddaughter, Renee, work full time outside the home. Son in-law Ron is semi-retired from his work in sales.

> I have a lot of company with Rene—but more than Rene, with Ron. He comes home two or three times a day. When I first moved here, I cut my thumb, almost to the bone. I had a knife that was dull, and I was cutting up a pot roast. I got so upset because I'm on Coumadin® [anticoagulation medicine].

> *I didn't call Pat. I called Ron. He said to put pressure on it, and just hold it there for about a half hour. I went next door because a nurse lives there, but she wasn't home. So I'm holding it with pressure—that's what he told me—and then it will stop. And it did. So, then Ron comes in, and makes sure that I'm not laying there somewhere.*

When working with your brothers and sisters, take this opportunity to draw on the diverse strengths of each. If one brother is more nocturnal, perhaps he can spell the person who has been doing the daytime caregiving. You may have one sibling who passes a grocery store on her way to the parent's home. She could be responsible for picking up food staples.

### Communication among Siblings

Every successful caregiving task has to start with clear communication. Think about the issues and problems that you are about to discuss with your brothers and sisters. Start the conversations with some possible solutions, instead of exposing a problem that could end in a standoff between you and the others.

> *Our children? I think the three of them communicate together a lot. And, if one is going to come home and visit in April, maybe the next one will plan on another few months, and they'll come home for a short time. They've kind of handled that pretty well by themselves, and we pretty much kind of leave it up to them to come when they can, really. I sound like a "Miss Goodie-two-shoes," I know.*

> **—Dolores (pseudonym), 82**

Revisit past experiences that have been successful. Whether you and your brothers solve family problems through a teleconference or over a game of billiards, use the venue you find best. For some family members, e-mail or writing old-fashioned letters is the best way to discuss difficult problems. Lustbader and Hooyman (1994) suggest creating a timeline for tasks to be completed. Nothing is etched in concrete, especially in circumstances where the ailing parent may have a debilitating disease and when a parent's length of life is quickly coming to an end.

The following letter is from an adult daughter named Nancy to her four siblings. By outlining her views on the next steps to take once her mother is released from the hospital, she hopes for the best possible outcome. Nancy is the only child who lives in the same city as her ailing 82-year-old mother.

*Dear Bloodlings,*

*I guess the older I get the simpler I like things to get; the less I like to struggle or put up a fight. I don't get a rush from a challenge like I used to. Now I tend to not only look both ways before I cross the street, but to look down to make sure I'm not stepping into a pothole—or worse.*

*I've been feeling rotten for weeks now, and I'm not going to make it any more dramatic than that. (Our sister) Mare came into town on the tail end of it, and it's been exhausting just to watch everything she's jumped into and accomplished since she's been here. Makes me dizzy. I have to stay in at least through today, and I've been absolutely no help to her at all. I'm so glad she's here.*

*Being temporarily incapacitated with this virus, plucked away from daily stressors that otherwise occupy my mind, has given me a chance to make several profound observations about my brothers and sister and the situation that's facing us all right now. I see that I am richly blessed to be one of five siblings who care so greatly not only for one another, but for our mother. I've seen reactions to this situation come from the core of our souls, not a single "whatever."*

*The raw talents God has blessed each of us with are being hauled out onto the table and exposed without protective shields for all to see, and they are many and magnificent. And we are vulnerable while they are exposed.*

*I felt a tremendous relief when Kareem and I made the decision to move Mom into our house upon discharge from the hospital. But after that decision was made, I realized that she would be living with me only because she was unable to live unattended and would need me to toilet her, prepare her meals, and provide sitters for her when I couldn't be here. Twenty-four-hour care equals nursing home. Although it felt like the right thing to do and I was more than willing to do it, I was wrestled down on this one. As it turns out, that scenario is not the one we have right now, anyway. She's able to do just about as much physically now as she could before she got sick (which isn't all that much, but at least is at a functional level).*

*Lying here and mulling, mulling, more and more the same thing keeps rising to the surface of the sludge pond. Mom is so happy to be coming home. She is a different person: (1) She's been through a life-altering experience and (2) she's now on Prozac. We must be the ones to make the decisions in her life now, and she is aware of that and that's okay with her. Our decisions must be wise, and we must be gentle with her in making them. Her health is fragile. The episode that put her in the hospital will not be an isolated one; being in the business of caring for geriatric patients, I can tell you that, statistically, patients with vascular disease who suffer from ulcers and colitis are "frequent fliers" for hospitalization. She will be in and out of the hospital, each time coming out progressively weaker.*

*Our (home health) agency knows we will be taking her on as a "lifer" this time, not just for a few months; she will be seen several times a week by a home health nurse, a physical therapist, and a CNA for bathing and hygiene. That's a lot of activity going on in her apartment, a lot of people becoming a part of her life from now on. With all this care she may make it much longer between hospitalizations than she would otherwise, and her care team will become a sort of family to her.*

*So I guess that I believe Mom already lives in an "assisted living facility." Mare and I will need the next few weeks to see how functional she will become on her own (that is, can she be left unattended at night?). With the home health service (which is paid 100% by Medicare) providing intermittent visits throughout the week and our caregiver's supplemental daily visits, I think staying in her apartment until the day that nursing home placement is necessary is the best plan both practically and financially.*

*Leaving her in her apartment will lift a burden from me as her primary caregiver—I've been taking care of all her outside needs thus far without a problem. She'll now have a wheelchair for making transportation outside her home easier. And leaving her in her apartment will eliminate the tremendous stress of moving. She wants only to be at home with her cat, "The Andy Griffith Show," and "Keeping Up Appearances."*

*So that's my observation. Given all our talents and abilities to think things through, how shall we know the best thing to do? Shall we make this decision as in a conclave of the Cardinals, writing down our thoughts on what's best for our mother on a piece of paper and burning each piece, seeing which is blessed by the Holy Spirit and produces white smoke? I recognize my blessing that I am your sister.*

XXOO, N

*Siblings Sharing Financial Responsibilities*

When siblings are making monetary contributions to assist in a parent's financial shortfall, resentment can surface about how the money is being allocated. Caregivers are more likely to provide financial assistance to their parents than adult children who are not caregivers, according to the report from The Center on an Aging Society, Georgetown University (2005). In one family that I worked with, I witnessed disagreement over how many paper goods were being purchased by the paid caregiver. In another, one adult son tried desperately to negotiate a lower price for a used commode for his mother.

Not only does a family conference have to take place before the monies are contributed and dispersed for the parent's care, but an accounting should be available on a quarterly basis to all siblings. Periodic reviews of the contributions and expenditures should also be agreed upon.

*My son and daughter are separated by miles—one in California, the other in New Orleans. They are not close sentimentally. He has been disgusted and disinterested with her because of financial matters. They talk to each other, but they don't go out of their way to see each other.*

*When I got so sick two summers ago, my daughter left work, came to Chicago, and stayed for a week. Then my granddaughter took over. She found out the diagnosis, spoke with the doctor, and transferred all information to my son and daughter-in-law before they arrived.*

*Then my son came and he was the one that took over. I was so amazed at this whole thing. At first he called me every single day, sometimes twice a day. Now he calls every two or three days. I would never have believed that my son's concern was this great. He had such a strong sentiment of sympathy. It surprised me—that he had become this close to me, and that he would feel this strongly about what had happened to me.*

*My grandson would visit and call every day. I have the most marvelous family. I would never have known this closeness had I not been this ill.*

—Charlotte S., 92

## When The Team Falls Apart

Sisters and brothers who have become estranged over parental care issues are most likely at odds over either money, power, resentment, or control—or all four. Unfortunately, many of these battles are fueled by past resentment and disagreements that date back years before the aging parent needed help. Some sibling and aging-parent battles become so serious that they end up as court cases resulting in bitterness and expensive legal bills. So many of these disagreements start over trivial matters and misunderstanding.

Chief Judge Milton Mack, of the Wayne County Probate Court in Detroit, said in an article for the National Advisory Council for Long Term Care Insurance (2005), "You sit up on the bench, listen, and just shake your head at what goes on. You are dealing with people who are educated and professional with good jobs but can't keep their eyes on what's important." Mack, who hears about 400 guardianship cases a year, says most are trouble-free. But about 10% of the cases become sibling power struggles played out before the judge, as he says, "ranging from not agreeing with one another on what's best for the parent to one sibling assaulting or threatening another."

## Keeping the Negotiations Alive by Bringing in a Mediator

One alternative to allowing adult children and their siblings to fall apart over disagreements about care is to call in help. Specialists in family counseling can facilitate the conference between siblings. The counselor will gather all participating family members together, assess the problem, and help work out a viable solution. Counselors can be found through the following agencies:

American Counseling Association
5999 Stevenson Ave. Alexandria, VA 22304
800-347-6647/800-473-2329 (fax)
703-823-6862 (TDD)

Family Counseling and Consulting, Inc.
www.family-counseling.com

National Board for Certified Counselors, Inc. and Affiliates
3 Terrace Way, Suite D
Greensboro, NC 27403-3660
336-547-0607/336-547-0017 (fax)
nbcc@nbcc.org <nbcc@nbcc.org>

*Action Steps*

- In every action, decision and battle that you wage with your siblings, remember that your first concern is to do what is best for your aging parent.
- This has been stated in other chapters, but will be repeated again. When possible, involve ailing parents in every decision about their care. Don't make decisions by sibling committee without your parent's vote.
- Now is not the time to let old grievances or rivalries come to the surface. What was in the past, should stay in the past.
- If you are the sibling who sees the parent the least, perhaps because you live out of town, don't arrive with "all-knowing" advice before you can fully assess how your brothers and sisters have been handling the care management duties.
- If another sibling has taken the lead in care management, offer to spell that brother or sister on a regular basis. Depression and caregiver burnout, although not always obvious, exist in the majority of family care situations.
- Other siblings may not know how to ask for help. Be proactive and anticipate your other family members' needs.
- If problems have arisen between siblings because of your parent's financial matters, it may be time to call in an impartial professional to help solve the problems.

Cherish the quality time you and your siblings have left with your ailing parent. At the same time, continue to build and nurture your relationships with your sisters and brothers. In some cases, an ailing parent's condition will bring estranged siblings together. Be proactive, instead of reactive about compliments, criticism, and advice. Take advantage of every positive moment. Remember that team building means treasured partnerships and tightening the ties that bind.

# CHAPTER 12

# Where Is the Love?

*"Let me know if you hear anything. I won't be in court this afternoon."*

—An adult son's response to a call that his 94-year-old father had just been rushed to the hospital with severe chest pains. The son was a circuit court judge, and worked just a few blocks from the hospital.

## When Love Falls Away from the Giving Side of Care

Those of us who work on the professional side of care management rarely hear both sides of the story when a family member chooses to take *no* responsibility for an ailing parent. More often than not, we don't get the facts about what led up to the family's estrangement. The following is another example of love and compassion taking a back seat to the provision of care. This directive came to me from an adult daughter who had moved her mother into our retirement community. "There is no love between me and my mother. I look after her for purely custodial care."

Yet the dutiful daughter visited her mother several times a week, provided for her every need, and was an advocate for the best possible care. This scenario turned out to be the first of many I witnessed by adult children or relatives about the love, or lack of love, at the center of their relationships with their parents.

This chapter focuses on family relationships, including estranged family members; "prodigal" sons and daughters who don't show up until the time of, or after, the parent's death; and the stress of the "good child" who provides care 24 hours a day, 7 days a week. What the fighting and resentment may all be about is covered in detail. Sometimes family members back away to the point of neglect. This chapter provides resources and direction about calling in the authorities. Action steps at the end of the chapter suggest strategies for intervention, coping, and healing.

Dan, who suffers from Parkinson's disease, is 85. He has four adult children, but is only close to his son. He became estranged from his daughters following Dan's bitter divorce more than 27 years ago. "My other children won't talk to me because of the divorce being so difficult, and my [former] wife has got them [convinced] that it's my fault, and there's not too much I can do about it." Dan describes the anger that still exists between his former wife and daughters and himself as "terrible."

As in Dan's situation, events that have happened in years past may have soured the relationships between parents and their children. As aging parents transition through the last chapters of their lives, the boundary lines of love and care become more clearly defined. For some family members, at the close of a parent's life there is healing. Others take their disputes to the grave.

Often families have experienced a falling-out over a divorce or over blended family arrangements where an aging parent has remarried. Many times, if a man has remarried a younger woman who the adult children resent, there is much family discord during the final months and days of the father's life. Add in the dynamics of adult children and stepchildren, and the relationship mix becomes even more complicated.

### "Prodigal" Sons and Daughters

The adult child who has been estranged from the family, by distance or by emotional involvement, was introduced in the previous chapter, but the topic is revisited here because the intensity of the estrangement within the family context needs to be noted.

In many families, the child who remains distant and sometimes doesn't make an appearance until after the aging parent has died, is often the adult child that the parent cherishes most. The estrangement characteristics among family members can range from parents or adult children not speaking to each other to someone taking legal action with court orders issued for restraint.

For the adult child who has been doing most of the full-time caregiving, the arrival of the estranged brother, sister, or even former spouse can cause anger and frustration. If the possibility exists that communication can be opened up between the two family members who are estranged, they should meet on mutual ground at a time that is pleasant and appropriate for both. Should there be no opportunity for reconciliation, then the full-time caregiving individual should take this opportunity to take a break by turning over responsibility to the visiting sibling, and indulge in some quality private time.

### When Families Fall Out Over Money

In many families, the standoff between adult children and their parents or siblings is about money. Money can be either the great motivator or the great divider. The disharmony could be about an inheritance, or the child may perceive an inequity in the parent's monetary support of other siblings. An adult child may believe that the parents are wasting their money on trivial things. Or perhaps the aging relative has decided to not part with a dime for his or her own health care management.

When I worked as the executive director of a retirement community in Chicago, I often listened to the lament of one particular adult son, who was an only child, about his elderly father's financial holdings. Much to the son's chagrin, his father had designated a local charity to receive 100% of his life savings upon his death. When voluntarily disclosing this information to me, the son added, "I could really use a new car. I really need that money."

The best way to approach a problem is to confront it as a unified group that includes your ailing parent and other family members who are involved in the dispute. An open, honest discussion is the best route, but not always the most practical.

When your estrangement from your parent is about money, you and your other family members should consult a professional in the field about your options. Talk to lawyers, financial experts, and estate planners. If your parent's money is in a trust, arrange a meeting with the trust officer at the bank. These meetings may only produce information, not change. Be aware, however, that you may not receive the outcome that you would like.

> *So you can tell your children, or the children can tell their parents, there should be this connection which I fully believe in. I don't think that anything is more important. Life is empty without love, tenderness, compassion, caring, sharing and relating.*
>
> —Danny, 85

### Pulling Others into Troubled Waters

If there is a rift in your family, or if there is a relationship that is supposed to be kept a secret, don't pull professional staff members into the problems. Employees at long-term care facilities should never be asked to keep confidences about moral or inappropriate family issues. Keep it in the family. The only exception to this rule is if you or your family members are enlisting a social worker or psychologist to help the family work through its problems. In that case, the health care professionals will keep all information confidential.

## When Abuse or Neglect Enter the Mix

The United States Administration on Aging (AOA) has compiled some arresting statistics about elder abuse. Unfortunately, elder abuse is a very broad topic; however, the focus here is on neglect and types of abuse inflicted by family and caregivers. Consider this. According to a 1998 AOA report:

- Each year hundreds of thousands of older persons are abused, neglected, and exploited by family members.
- More than 551,011 persons aged 60 and over experienced abuse, neglect, or self-neglect (see below) in a 1-year period.
- Among known perpetrators of abuse and neglect, the perpetrator was a family member in 90% of cases.
- Two thirds of the perpetrators were adult children or spouses.

The National Center on Elder Abuse defines these seven areas as the major types of elder abuse:

1. Physical abuse
2. Sexual abuse
3. Emotional or psychological abuse
4. Neglect
5. Abandonment
6. Financial or material exploitation
7. Self-neglect

"Self-neglect" may be a term that is not as familiar when general references are made about abuse. Self-neglect is characterized as the behavior of an elderly person that threatens his or her own health or safety. Self-neglect generally manifests as a refusal or failure to provide oneself with adequate food, water, clothing, shelter, personal hygiene, medication (when indicated), and safety precautions. It can be a result of mental illness where an individual is incapable of providing care for himself.

When abuse of an elderly individual is detected and reported and there are no family members, or family members won't get involved, the state's public guardian will be called in. If a staff member of a health care facility or home care agency sees evidence of neglect or abuse regarding a dependent elderly resident or patient, it will be reported.

Similarly, if you should witness inappropriate behavior while you are at a physician's office, long-term care facility, a therapy session, or in a private setting, always report the incident to the proper authorities. In your community, or in your travels, if you come upon a senior who is living in squalor, or who exhibits visible signs of neglect, immediately contact the nearest social service agency or the local police.

### It's Dishonest/Cheating/Illegal

When adult children are handling their dependent parents' finances, they sometimes try to hide the net worth of their elders. On more than one occasion as a health care professional in the long-term care field, I have seen the family of a resident try to qualify their relative for public aid monies, even though they could well afford their care, or room and board. When I was a marketing director for a nursing home outside of Chicago, an adult daughter of a potential resident posed this question. "I would like my mother to go on public aid. How can I hide the fact that, in addition to her home here, she also owns a condo in Aspen? I don't want to have to sell it."

Who loses in this situation? Everybody. Trying to receive public aid funding when you have monetary resources cheats all of us (as taxpayers). It also jeopardizes aid for residents who truly qualify for those funds. Bottom line? It's illegal. Both children and their dependent parents run the risk of severe penalties, a criminal record for fraud, and possible jail time. Don't do it. Not only might you be caught, but also you are muddying up the system for those who really need monetary assistance.

Next, do not ask any of the professionals you deal with—lawyers, health care workers, and long-term care administrators—to help you with your plan. It's just wrong.

### Action Steps

- Whether the estrangement is between you and your ailing parent, or your parent and your siblings, get professional help. A health care professional, a counselor, clergy, or family doctor can help you see more clearly how to reduce the stress on your family relationships.
- If the estrangement between the aging parent and adult child is about money, consult a professional in the field about your options. Talk to lawyers, financial experts, trust officers, and estate planners. These meetings may produce only information, not change. Be prepared for the outcome. It may not be in your favor.
- Remember the creed introduced in an earlier chapter: "Giving in doesn't mean giving up." At times, you have to put your pride aside.

If you have to give in to another family member's wishes, keep in mind that your goal is to do the absolute best for your ailing family member.

- You are dealing with the "here and now." The past is in the past. Don't allow past rifts with siblings or broken promises with your loved one to make your situation more difficult. Sometimes elders become irritable to get attention as a result of loneliness.

If someone you care about is in imminent danger regarding abuse or neglect, call 911. Every state has a toll-free number to report or answer questions about elder abuse. The website is www.elderabusecenter.org or call the Eldercare Locator at 800-677-1116.

When you look up the definition of family in a dictionary, the first reference is to individuals united by bloodline and ancestry. A second definition states that a family is "a group of people united by certain convictions." Nowhere does it say that family members have to like each other. But the second definition about "family convictions" implies that in each family unit there is a common thread that binds the members together.

As professionals view family dynamics from the sidelines, it is difficult to know what went on in the family's history. When we observe elderly individuals and their families who are separated by hate and anger, it is difficult not to offer hope. Perhaps caregivers in fractured families can dig a little deeper to find a conviction that may foster hope for future reconciliation and peace.

*And that's what you could tell the (adult) children whose parents are growing old: "If you really love your parents, give them your love. They don't need somebody to give them money as much as they need somebody to … go to the store for them … to wash the dishes for them.*

*Call them on the phone every day, every other day, every third day. "Hi Mom. Hi Pop. How are you? What's doing? How are you getting along?" That's what you tell the children.*

—Dan, 85

# CHAPTER 13

# What About God? Is He Still Listening to Me at This Age?

*George was a devoted church member all his life. He continued to be actively involved in his congregation, even though he could no longer attend church services because of his physical challenges. He had become a master at computer graphics, so he made it his mission to create greeting cards for shut-ins and sent birthday cards to other parishioners.*

*His church community activities, however, represented a sharp contrast to George's personal faith. When asked if his relationship with God had changed since he had contracted amyotrophic lateral sclerosis (ALS), or Lou Gehrig's disease, he said, "Having ALS did not affect my religious beliefs. But, to be honest, I don't really believe in God."*

— George, 77

During the last chapters of life, elders face some of life's greatest challenges: disease, frailty, loss of independence, and ultimately death. A common thread that brings continuity to this journey for many is the sense of spirituality. As the poker game of life deals more physical ailments from its proverbial deck, many care receivers question whether God is still interested in their health and happiness at this stage in life, and how long they can stay in the game. For some elders, as they approach the end of life their sense of spirituality becomes more refined.

In the pages that follow, we will explore the spiritual journey that our aging elders are taking, and come to know why religious practices in later life take on new meaning. It's important that dependent elderly people keep the spiritual connection, especially if they have had to move out of their own homes. Strategies to make this connection appear later in the chapter.

Two different thoughts can present themselves when care receivers question their spirituality during the later part of life: (1) they may begin to doubt their faith because God hasn't taken away their pain, or (2) they can become significantly more aware of the hereafter because their time on earth is diminishing. Some care receivers want to cash in their chips regarding deals and promises they have made with God. Others rethink their previous end-of-life decisions regarding sustaining life or accepting death.

> *God help her, she suffers so much. I just want Him to take her out of her pain. That's my prayer every day.*

> **—Lou (pseudonym), primary caregiver to his 93-year-old wife**

During the first half of the 20th century, churches and synagogues were the backbone of communities. The church, for many, was the hub of social life. My parents met at the youth group at their Presbyterian church, courted and shared married life for 57 years. My friend Marilyn's parents, who were married for 63 years, met at Luther League, the youth organization at the Lutheran church where they worshiped.

The care receivers focused on in this book represent the generation who lived through World War II, and some who experienced the atrocities of the Holocaust first-hand in the name of religion. In the Depression era and until about 1970, it was acceptable to pray in public school classrooms, and religion was clearly defined.

In the United States, if elders of the Depression era were brought up with religion in the home, they most likely practiced Catholicism, Judaism, or Protestantism. These three dominant religions were at the core of spirituality for most of our aging parents and grandparents. In this century, as the world has become more multicultural, hundreds of other religions are practiced in our country.

> *I feel there is no scientific way to prove or disprove God's existence. There are so many Christian churches and so many other religions that have existed over the centuries that have claimed to be the truly ONE alone. Since there are so many religions, I think mankind must have a basic need for religion.*

> **—George, 77, who suffered from ALS**

There are many studies that suggest that older adults who attend religious services or who participate in spiritual activity such as prayer or meditation are likely to live longer. One research study of 1,931 older adults, published in the *American Journal of Public Health* (1999), indicates that those who regularly attend religious services have a lower mortality rate.

It is important for frail care receivers to feel that they have a place and a voice in their churches, especially if they are unable to attend services on a regular basis. Family members, especially family caregivers, need to take action to keep an elderly person's physical and emotional connection to a place of worship.

The spiritual community can provide an important network of support and friendship. Having parishioners or clergy come for visits or to bring communion can often lift the spirits of a shut-in. Some churches televise services for the homebound or have services available on audiocassettes. Action steps at the end of this chapter suggest ways that the homebound care receiver can be involved in the church, such as addressing cards or making calls from home.

### The Dependent Elderly: Closer to Heaven?

Chaplain Supervisor Noel Brown at Northwestern Memorial Hospital in Chicago doesn't hear as much about heaven as one would think from the elderly patients he visits. "Most folks who are near the end of their lives look at heaven as a place where they will be reunited with family and friends. But the majority don't think about it in religious terms. People are more occupied with the here and now. There aren't very many sermons that talk about the 'furniture of heaven' anymore."

> *There are no real conceptions of heaven or its singular hell ... I don't know that I would be happy in either one or the other. I'm sure there are times when there is a road or a path or something that you walk along to get into a situation. I hope I'm on that path toward heaven, but I know the people that I visualize as being in heaven might have been thrown out before they could get there, for traits that God says are wrong. They may or may not be. It's pretty hard to put yourself in the supreme point to know what is heavenly and what is devilish. It requires a more agile mind than I've got.*
>
> *For instance, there are groups of people that come to your house and knock on your door and want to tell you how to get to heaven, or how to live forever. They often are astonished by the fact that I don't want to live forever, and I'm not in any rush to get to heaven.*
>
> —Jimmy, 85

*Frailties and Human Suffering—Is God To Blame?*

Many of the dependent elderly experience physical suffering because they are stuck in a body that isn't cooperating. Some individuals suffer the excruciating daily pain of arthritis; others lose touch with a portion of the outside world through hearing or vision loss. For a generation who has grown up with a formal religious background, is it fair to blame a supreme being for life's ailments?

For the majority of the elderly residents that Chaplain Brown ministers to, there is no anger toward God regarding human infirmities. "By this stage, people have come to terms with their lives. The exceptions are those people who are still angry, since they have been angry all their lives. An individual's religious beliefs don't change during the last stage of life."

Dora, 88, had been a concert pianist all her life. A native of Port Arthur, Ontario, Dora came to Chicago as a young woman in her 20s to study music and made Chicago her home. Throughout her career she traveled the world as an accompanist to many world-famous musicians.

Today, because of a severe melanoma, Dora has no sight in one eye, and can detect only shadows in the other. She lives in an assisted living facility in Chicago. As an only child who never married, Dora doesn't have any relatives in the United States. She has hired paid caregivers who provide personal care several hours a day.

Dora doesn't feel she has suffered because of her loss of sight, and she harbors no bitterness in her heart toward God. "Look what the Lord went through. No, I have a faith. We're in the hands of the Lord, and the Lord guides us. When I think about my own life and the things that have happened, I could not have made them happen. Some higher power has to be behind it. What guides our life? The Lord."

A determined woman about her faith, Dora has no time for people who are ambivalent about God. "You're either with the Lord or you're not. Give thanks to the Lord every single day for your life. Truly, the way my life has worked out, it has been led by a higher power."

*I'm not afraid of dying. I figure everyone has to go at some time.*

—Charlotte Z., 94

*Your Life is Getting Shorter, Are You Closer to God?*

As people transition through their final chapter of life, do they establish a new covenant with their God? Many people continue their relationship with their Lord in whatever form they had all their lives. "It's a chicken-and-egg question," according to Chaplain Brown. "The way they are is how they believe, and the way they believe is the way they are."

*As her elder years have progressed, Rose has felt closer to her God. "That's been going on for many years. It's really something that we don't have enough time to prepare for. Today, tomorrow, it's always gone. If you are not prepared to meet your Maker, you have failed."*

*Rose has also made it her goal to increase her private time with God through prayer. "I said, 'God, I have the time'. If I can't give a half hour or so to God, life isn't worth it. I can't go to church because I would be bumping around with my walker. My relationship with God is closer. You can just visualize it. He's going to be there to welcome you. I wish I would have known better to do a couple of things in my life. I was already on the right track [toward God]."*

—Rose, 93, lives in a nursing home in Wisconsin

### Making Agreements with and Demands of God

Do people barter with God for more time to live, or to live better lives? "People who feel that their life is over want God to take them now," Chaplain Brown says. "There are people who will themselves to stay alive until a certain event happens—the wedding of a favorite grandchild or the birth of a great-grandchild. Many people make promises to be faithful so that they can be alive for that special event."

In the book *Soulful Aging, Ministry through the Stages of Adulthood* (2001), contributing author John Yungblut describes the aging process by which a person starts to disconnect from God. "As we age, it is important to realize that the many kinds of darkness we know can be opportunities for the deepening of love. Without such support and assurance, we will seek escape, suffer unnecessary pain, or fall into despair. For example, one kind of darkness that I have heard expressed by those in the last years of a long life is a sense of being abandoned by God. The light is dimming and going out, and they cannot find God's presence in the darkness. Older persons have expressed this to me in different ways, but one component is often a readiness to die and the inability to find any purpose for one's life."

Yungblat speaks from professional and personal experience as an Episcopal minister for 20 years, and as a person who suffers from Parkinson's disease. "It is possible, on one level, to distinguish spiritual darkness from the darkness of depression and grief. Spiritual darkness is often accompanied by several signs: peace at a level deeper than the surface agitation and distress, a desire for spiritual experiences and a longing to pursue them even though usual forms no longer give satisfaction, and good functioning in the other areas of one's life."

At times, discussing spirituality and religious beliefs presents some awkward moments between frail elderly people and their family caregiver or their paid professional care provider. Caregivers may become uncomfortable in talking about spirituality, or the "hereafter," especially if the care receiver is suffering or close to death.

It is important to allow care receivers to express their thoughts, and to be respectful of the ailing family members' beliefs. Wendy Lustbader, M.S.W. suggests good listening skills, and the encouragement of expression, with the hope that through this process, the caregiver can try to understand how the care receiver is bearing their circumstances. *In Taking Care of the Caregivers*, (Lustbader, Hooyman, 1994), the authors suggest dialog that will deflect probing questions about the caregiver's beliefs without being disrespectful of the care receiver's beliefs: "Mom, I am not sure where I stand on all of this, but it's good to hear your reflections."

*The Power of Personal Prayer*

In the book *Soulful Aging* (2001), authors Henry Simmons and Mark Peters offer a visit plan for clergy who minister to residents in nursing homes. They reveal a disparity between the needs of the residents and the perceptions of the clergy.

> *A study of the perception of needs in three long-term care facilities compares the residents' understanding of their needs for pastoral care and that of their pastors. The residents said unanimously that what helped them move through impact and recoil to reorganization and adaptation of spirituality was personal prayer. The pastoral ministers, on the other hand, thought the need was for communal worship, for collective activities.*
>
> *While both ministers and residents agreed on the need for reassurance, for the re-creation of a meaningful life, and for a personal relationship with God, the residents reported that these needs were met through private and personal spiritual activity and deeper involvement in the internal side of spirituality.*

*Relocation and Spiritual Disconnect*

Simmons and Peters (2001) also studied the impact of the transition to a nursing home, and how a new resident's personal prayer rituals are disrupted. "How specific is this moment in the life of a nursing home resident, and how personal is the struggle to make a successful transition? People will say that they have prayed personal prayers, but in some measure, familiar people, familiar places, and familiar weekly rhythms of prayer have supported their prayers. Now the places the resident prayed are no longer their places of prayer; and the self who prayed there is no longer the same self. The resident cannot go home again, physically or spiritually. There is a sense of uprootedness that needs to be articulated forthrightly. Only when it is named is it fair to add that it is possible to begin to pray again in this new old age."

*Action Steps*

- For the care receiver who has been separated from his or her own parish, or has stopped attending regular worship services, it is important to keep them involved. Some churches and synagogues call on shut-ins to have them help address cards and help with mailings. The housebound elderly can also make phone calls to other persons who are in need.
- If your elderly parent lives out of town, call his or her local church about volunteers who could bring communion or Bible study to your parent. Find out what church or temple groups your parent used to attend, and inquire about visits from other members of the group.
- If the care receiver is unable to attend services, have a volunteer or clergyperson visit. The visitor should bring along the weekly church bulletin and offer communion where appropriate.
- Encourage your loved one to stay connected spiritually, even though they are unable to physically make it to their church.
- Communication should be open about the elder's beliefs. It is important that the care receiver's feelings of self worth are not compromised because of physical separation from a familiar place of worship.
- If your loved one has spiritual beliefs that differ from those of the rest of the household, encourage all family members to be respectful of each other's beliefs and opinions.
- Some churches offer Bible study groups that are accessible to those in need. If your elderly loved one can't get out, volunteer to have a Bible study group meet at your home.

Whether elderly relatives have Alzheimer's disease or are dependent on you as a caregiver because of limited mobility, their spiritual needs must to be included in their care plan. Just as you take action to fulfill physical, social, and emotional needs, the spiritual component must be pursued. The spiritual tasks could include finding a house of worship that is accessible to someone in a wheelchair or providing a hymnal to homebound people so that they can participate in televised religious services. Keeping loved ones connected spiritually will bring them a higher quality of life and an increased sense of community and purpose.

# CHAPTER 14

# The End of the Road:
# Death as Life's Final Chapter

*Dying is a very dull and dreary affair. And my advice to you is to have nothing whatever to do with it.*

—William Somerset Maugham

A caregiver's own emotional reaction to the death of a loved one after a long illness comes as a surprise to many family care providers. Although many who have provided care and support realize that their family member is now released from pain, the caregivers are sometimes shocked into a numbness that their own caregiving duties are over. Some describe this feeling as "swimming under water." Even care providers who have traveled a very long road with their ailing relatives feel they are unprepared for the finality of death.

In this chapter, caregivers will learn about their feelings of "losing their 'job' after all this time." Grief, remorse, guilt, and family dynamics are also explored. Tips on communication with children about death are shared. One brother of a suicide victim advises family members to, "tell everyone you know," about the death. He coaches others to solicit support from "their immediate world" at this difficult time in their lives.

There are many studies about the anxiety and stress levels of caregivers prior to and following the death of their care recipient. The Alzheimer's Disease Education & Referral Center published findings from a study showing that caregivers who exhibited high levels of depressive symptoms while caring for their relative with dementia experienced much lower rates of clinical depression after their loved one's death (2001). These studies showed significant declines in depression after the year following the death.

This chapter also provides an explanation of advance directives, including living will, health care power of attorney, and organ donation information. Common questions about hospice care are also answered. Can your loved one stay at home under hospice care? Are you allowed to call an ambulance if hospice is involved? Who pays for hospice? Action steps in this chapter help readers make decisions about what to expect at the time of death, final arrangements, and the healing process that follows a death.

### The Ties That Bind

*Shielding Each Other from News*   Individuals who have accepted the inevitability of their imminent death often try to protect their family members from the obvious. In turn, family caregivers also make efforts to shield their dying loved ones from knowing their final fate. Sue Black, RN, BSN, now retired from the Fox Valley Hospice in Geneva, Illinois, encountered many situations where family members tried to protect each other. "I would walk into a home. The family would say, 'Mother is dying but don't tell her.' I would go into her room and she would say, 'I am dying, but don't tell my family.' It would be my job to get them to communicate together. When it worked, it was wonderful. When it did not work, we had to approach things in a totally different way."

The best way to get answers is to ask the right questions in a sensitive and loving way. Ask loved ones if they would like to share what lies ahead. Explain to your parents that you are prepared to make this journey with them, and that your hope would be that would not try to shield you from the inevitable. Discuss how you would like to partner with them to provide the best options for their care. Let them know that you need all the facts before you can offer the best help.

### Talking to Children About a Loved One's Death

> *I never thought I'd live this long. Never. So, I don't know why. Sometimes I think it's for punishment. I don't know. Something that I didn't do right in my life or something. That's why I'm living this long. Because a lot of times I feel like the kids wonder, 'Gee, when is she going to go?'*
>
> —Estelle, 94

As adults, we are conditioned to accept the inevitability of life's end. Although we grieve, we had always expected that we would outlive our parents. Young children don't understand what death is all about and they haven't developed coping skills.

When a grandparent or elderly relative dies, we need to acknowledge that the child's heart is hurting, and understand that grief takes on a different tone at different ages. Help children through this grief journey by explaining death in a realistic way, and encourage them to cry, talk—and laugh and play—if that is how they can express their grief. Children should be told that the death was not their fault, and that it is part of the life cycle. It is important, too, that you calm children's fears about losing other people in their lives.

Help your child understand the ritual of the funeral service or Shiva, and talk about which family members will be participating in services. Let the child's teacher and parents of friends know that the child is going through the grieving process.

### What Physicians Share with Patients and Families about Death

Physicians are directed to share only as much information about their patient's condition as the patient is willing to know. As outlined in *TAKE CARE! Magazine* (Fall 2004), this mandate comes from a 2000 American Medical Association program entitled, "End-of-Life Care." The program advises physicians to:

- Assess what patients already know about their conditions.
- Ask patients how much they want to know about their conditions.
- Provide them with only as much information as they want to know.

By following these guidelines the doctor is acting in an ethical and professional manner. For example, if the patient wants to hear very little news unless it is good news about hope, then under the AMA directive, the physician should share only news that is honest about hope, as limited as it may be.

The directive described above, combined with new laws about medical confidentiality, leaves families with few sources about the condition of their ailing relative, unless the care receiver himself discloses the information. Respecting the patient's wishes is first and foremost.

Now that this fairly one-sided explanation of disclosure has been presented, a family member may feel left out of the loop about their loved one's prognosis. You, as the caregiver, may also feel at a loss about how much time your loved one has left, and how you are expected to cope. In the same article in *TAKE CARE! Magazine* (Fall 2004), clinical psychologist Dr. Barry Jacobs suggests, "By focusing on contingencies rather than prognoses, you may still wind up having the conversation that you would like while allowing your parent to face his final struggle in the manner he has chosen."

### The Hospice Journey of Fred and Becky

*Narrative by Hospice Volunteer Sue Black*   Fred was an independent man who had a brusque way of keeping people at an emotional distance when he chose to. He was dying of cancer. His voice was strong and loud as he sat perched atop his orange chair. Fred made the chair himself; he could breathe better sitting higher. And from this higher point in the room, Fred directed the activity in his living room. When he stood, his shoulders drooped and sometimes his head reached downward. But in his chair, he was "King of the Apartment," a position we tried to keep him in until his death.

Fred and his wife, Becky, shared a small apartment. Within the apartment, the center of his universe was Fred's massive desk. On it were tapes piled high, several tape recorders, many envelopes, a full ashtray, more cigarettes, brown medicine containers, a dial telephone, a coffee cup, and a glass of iced tea. There was a small blackboard on the wall with important telephone numbers on it. Looking back, I knew somehow that I'd really made it when my name and telephone number appeared on that board.

When I came to visit the first time, I found these two people struggling to make some sense out of what Fred called, "the doctor's death sentence." Fred explained, "Seven years ago the doctor told me I had three months to live. I guess God doesn't want me and the devil won't have me."

The overwhelming struggle I faced from the first day we met was not being able to get Fred's pain under better control. We tried one medication after another, yet nothing ever worked longer than 4 or 5 days. Fred's pain interrupted my thoughts when I was fixing meals, when I was scrubbing the floor, when I awoke during the night, and when I was on vacation. I met him in pain and he died in pain. Most of my patients had had little pain; I still feel Fred's.

Those two special people, who subsisted on disability and food pantry staples, drew me back each day like magnets. They shared their hopes and dreams, frustrations and nightmares. One day we talked about all the motels they had shared. We laughed together, cried together, shared recipes, drank iced tea, and loved each other. Fred would frequently ask, "Can't you stay a little longer?" And I always found myself owing my babysitter a little more on the days I visited Fred.

Fred touched the very roots of my soul, and because of him I will never be the same person again. I truly believe it was a once-in-a-lifetime experience. It was a relationship without pretenses, without masks. Each of us was able "to be." Fred said, "Don't ever apologize for who you are, what you've become, or where you live. You're one of our kind!"

*Emotions of the Dying: Independence, Anger, Control*

So many of the interviewees featured here found that giving up control of their lives, and becoming a burden to families was their biggest concern. Rev. Clarence R. Kelley, chaplain, Horizon Hospice and Palliative Care in Chicago said, "For geriatric patients, there is their need to remain in control as much as possible. That seems to be the biggest stigma about having to depend on others. There is a need not to worry other family members. They will say, 'I've lived my life; they have to live their life. They have children; they have responsibilities.' They don't want to infringe on their families with what they are going through. Don't want to bother the families. They want to let them live their lives."

There is also the desire by geriatric hospice patients to become released from their pain. Rev. Kelley said, "There are those who will say, 'I would rather die than live like this.' There is the piece about not wanting to suffer, or 'Why won't God just let me die?'"

Issues regarding control and independence during the stages of dying often mirrored how they were handled during a person's life, according to retired hospice nurse Sue Black. "I found that people died as they lived. Strong, take-charge men usually fought very hard when they were dying. They hated to give up that 'control' they had spent developing all their working lives. So many women were the nurturers of their individual families. They found it difficult to give up that role."

A dying person's personal faith plays a key role in how death is perceived, according to Black. "I found that a person's acceptance of death was often tied to his or her concept of religion or spirituality. People who believed there was an afterlife often accepted their condition more easily, because they felt they were going to a better place. People without such a foundation wanted to eke out all they could with the time remaining."

> *I am telling you this very candidly, and very truthfully: I would like to go to sleep one night and not get up in the morning. I can't stand the suffering. I have had plenty of suffering, all of the pills, and the heart, and with this and with that.*

> **—Danny, 85, suffering with Parkinson's disease**

*Acceptance or Denial*

Many individuals whose lives are controlled by debilitating diseases that will soon result in death would choose to hasten their own passing.

Northwestern Hospital Chaplain Supervisor Noel Brown explains, "While people don't necessarily make deals with God, when they feel their life is over, they want God to take them now."

> *I really didn't think about this stage of my life that much. I did hope that I would not be incapacitated for a long time and wouldn't be in uncontrollable pain.*

—George G., 77, suffering with ALS

Denial is the first stage of the death process for many, according to Horizon Hospice chaplain Rev. Kelley, "In dealing with their diagnosis and then prognosis, those patients who are in denial think that if they do the right thing—eat right, or change their lifestyle, the diagnosis could change." Acceptance replaces denial once the physical body starts to change. Rev Kelly says, "They move to a place of acceptance once their physical appearance changes. Now they know it is happening and can see it."

## A Hiatus from Death

In rare situations, patients are discharged from hospice care because their physical bodies have shown strong enough improvement to no longer be actively dying. Rev. Kelly had one patient to whom he ministered who was discharged from hospice care after 3 months. "This patient was in her 80s and had been in the hospital for quite some time. Her sister decided to take her home and feed her 'old Southern-style' foods including greens and a lot of different vegetables. The sister also had some special rubbing oil that she claimed was very good for the bones. The home remedies seemed to work for this particular patient."

## Hanging On

In many situations, people whose death is imminent have hung on to life to celebrate a certain event such as a grandchild's wedding or to reconcile with a loved one. They may even "postpone" their deaths until they can see a certain family member. In my own family, as my grandfather was dying of cancer, he chose to hang onto life a few days longer until his younger son was released from the hospital. Rev. Kelley cited one example of an elderly mother whose death was imminent. She willed herself to live a while longer until her son could be released from prison to come to her bedside. Her children told her, "Mom, everyone is here." And then she expired.

*Letting Go* Medical professionals and clergy who minister to the dying believe that people can will their physical bodies to expire. Due to the nature of the assumption, however, little, if any, data substantiates this idea. There are, however, many examples of people who have been observed to 'shut down' their physical bodies. "At some point, the person has the control to be able to tell the body, 'that's that', according to Rev. Kelley. "We need all of our emotional capabilities to keep us going. One's psychological perspective can bring about changes in one physiologically. You get physical responses from psychological situations. They are able to tell their bodies, 'I am ready.'"

### Respecting Your Loved One's Wishes

*Advance Directives*   Determining what steps should be taken regarding end-of-life issues for a family member will be an efficient task if your loved one has provided personal advance directive information. These documents should include, but are not limited to, a living will, durable power of attorney for health care, and organ donation documentation if desired.

- The living will document states an individual's intentions regarding medical care and life sustaining measures that he or she wants taken in the event that they become incapacitated.
- The durable power of attorney for health care allows the individual to name someone to speak on his behalf about medical decisions and life sustaining care if he is unable to speak for himself.
- Organ donation documents state your loved one's desire to donate his organs after he dies for research and for transplant purposes.

Several highly visible court cases have been played out in the media because specific individuals have not made their end-of-life wishes known, and families aren't sure about what measures to take. As a result, family members, medical professionals, and people with political interests join the fray to influence the decisions.

### Respecting a Wish About a Funeral

When Roma's (pseudonym) mom died suddenly of cancer, she hadn't made specific funeral plans for herself. Her mother's one wish, however, was that her adult children not spend a lot of money on her burial.

Her children respected their mother's wishes to be cremated, but when it came time to bury her ashes, the children were shocked at the costs of a simple burial. "My mother would have been mortified to find out that we would have to spend thousands of dollars to open the grave, put the ashes in a vault, and pay again for the services of burial. All this expense for a simple burial."

Roma and her siblings came up with a simple plan and carried it out. On the designated day, all of the adult children gathered at the cemetery plot. They had made no arrangements with the cemetery for the grave to be opened.

Instead, Roma and her brothers and sisters had brought along a bed of flowers to the cemetery. Each adult child dug a little hole above the grave, poured a cup full of ashes into the hole, placed a flower into the dirt in the hole, and covered the base of the flower. The children continued this ritual until all of the flowers had been planted.

Was this a legal burial procedure? Is this an act that other families should pursue? Maybe not. But Roma's mother's wishes about having a low-cost funeral were granted.

### Hospice Care

*Comfort and Compassion*   Although hospice care has been around in the United States since 1974, there is still a lot of mystery about its purpose. Hospice services are provided to an individual to maximize the quality of the remaining life through the provision of palliative or comfort care. These types of comfort therapies control the symptoms and minimize the negative effects of intervention.

Enrollment in hospice care can happen when the individual and his or her physician have determined that there is no hope for recovery. The usual time frame for life expectancy is to live 6 months or less; however, many hospice patients exceed that time span. Patients in a hospice program are reviewed over time to determine whether they should continue under hospice care.

When an individual gives his consent for hospice services, it doesn't mean giving up. However, interventions such as cardiopulmonary resuscitation (CPR), feeding tubes, and antibiotics for recurrent infections will no longer be used. A person's religious beliefs and cultural rituals should be reviewed when an individual is admitted to a hospice program. Hospice care provides a team of health care professionals, including a chaplain, who come in to provide comfort care and pain management. Other benefits include:

- Continuing care from a dedicated health care team committed to meeting the patient's and family's needs.
- A primary nurse assigned to each patient. The nurse visits regularly and coordinates the other professionals and volunteers. Families are able to call this nurse on a 24-hour on-call basis when there are questions.
- Reduced medical costs. Medicare includes a benefit that pays for hospice.
- Hospice services can also provide for medical equipment, such as hospital bed, wheelchair, oxygen, walker, etc. in the home.
- Self-determination regarding treatment and location of delivery.

- Respite services to give the family a break.
- Quality of life and a natural, dignified death.

Having a hospice nurse who acts as the liaison between the family and the other professional health care workers is a wonderful benefit. When my own parents were under hospice care, our hospice nurse was called on many times to help us understand each step of the dying process. She was able to translate technical medical information into terms that could be understood by everyone involved in my parents' care. Even after the death of each parent, the hospice nurse was able to walk us through the steps of what to do immediately after the death occurred. From a personal perspective, having her there in a professional capacity helped us get through many of the difficult tasks.

> *This year I can't seem to get in the mood to compose a Christmas letter. My niece wrote she was in Christmas denial. I feel that way. Although I think the powers-that-be were premature in qualifying me for the hospice program, I have been fortunate to get assistance from the hospice crew. I would like to find a way to expedite, to hasten my death. I've gotten literature from the Hemlock Society. But their method for ending one's life seems to me difficult to carry out, involving putting a plastic bag over one's head. I think total fasting would be better. In 1 to 2 weeks, it's over.*

—George, 76

To individuals who are unfamiliar with hospice care, there are some general misconceptions about the use of medications and medical procedures for hospice patients. If there is an emergency where immediate medical attention is needed, such as a fall resulting in broken bones, or a severe reaction to medication, these occurrences will be treated even though the patient is terminal. Antibiotics and other medicines will be administered to clear up infections such as urinary track infections that will cause short-term discomfort.

In reference to calling an ambulance for someone receiving hospice care, the first call should be to the 24-hour on-call hospice nurse. He or she can then determine if the emergency services are needed, and expedite getting the proper help.

*Finding Support*

When your loved one's death is imminent, try as much as you can to formulate a plan that will take you through the next 6 months. Although that seems like a painstaking assignment in your darkest hour, it could prove to be the foundation that keeps you going.

*Often I found the people who were dying to be the strength of the entire group. I was there not to support them, but to help their families to deal with the impending death and the aftermath.*

—**Sue, retired hospice nurse**

Another strategy to help you gain support and help during your grieving process is to communicate to everyone you can that you have had a death in the family. During a seminar I attended about grief counseling, the lecturer identified himself as a "suicide survivor" because he was the brother of a suicide victim. He stressed the importance of telling everyone you know about your relative's death, so that your inner and outer circles of support will help buoy you through this wave of grief. He went on to say that, unlike his sister, who told two co-workers she need a couple of days off for a funeral; the lecturer told his friends, co-workers, neighbors, and acquaintances about his brother's death. As a result, the young man had almost 100 loving people come to his brother's funeral to offer their support. Asking for help and support during your time of grief is critical.

### Understanding the Caregiver-Job Loss

A second factor that must be included in the 6-month plan mentioned above is tasks and assignments to take the place of the caregiver's job. Many caregivers find their newfound "freedom" a burden. Instead of being busy every minute as a family caregiver, many care providers find themselves at a loss once their dependent elderly relative dies. Transitioning back into a social life can be intimidating for the caregiver.

As part of taking care of yourself during the grieving process, make a list of all the positive tasks that you contributed to the care of your family member during his final days. Don't let yourself get caught up in the guilt mantra of "what ifs." "What if we had waited to go into hospice?" "What if we had tried one more experimental therapy?" Recognize that you did the best job you could do. Your loved one's passing was made better because he had you on his team.

### Action Steps

- Talk to dying loved ones about your role in their journey. Find out if they are willing to discuss the full nature of their illness, and their wishes about their deaths.
- Know where to find your family member's documentation about advance directives.
- Explore hospice options.

- Talk with children about death as part of life. Calm their fears about other family members' dying and explain the grieving and funeral rituals.
- As the family caregiver, formulate a 6-month plan that will fall into place upon the death of your aging parent. This plan will help with the transition after the caregiving role is over.
- Don't let yourself get caught up in feelings of guilt or remorse over interventions or tasks that could have made the dying process easier.
- Know that you did your best.

Closing life's last chapter is a painful task. Family caregivers are faced with a host of difficult decisions in the days leading up to their relative's death, and after the death. Value the discussions with your dying family member, and other members of the family. Make a concerted effort with children to explain the dynamics of your loved one's final days.

Be good to yourself. No one is capable of making perfect decisions. In death, as in life, cherish every single moment when you are able to make a good connection with your dying loved one.

# References

Alzheimer's Disease Education and Referral Center (2001). Research to Help Families and Caregivers. Progress Report. Retrieved May 30, 2005 from http://www.alzheimers.org/pr01-02/15.htm.

American Society on Aging (2000). The Sandwich Generation: Work/Life Balance of Child and Elder Caregiving, Demographics, Statistics. Retrieved May 5, 2002 from www.familycaregiversonline.

Avadian, B. (2002). *Finding the Joy in Alzheimer's Disease*, North Star Books.

Carter, R. and Golant, S.K. (1995). *Helping Yourself Help Others: A Book for Caregivers*. New York: Times Books.

Center on an Aging Society, Georgetown University (2005). Adult Children: The Likelihood of Providing Care for an Older Parent. Data Profile, Number 2, May 2005. Retrieved on June 11, 2005 from http://hpi.georgetown.edu/agingsociety/pdfs/CAREGIVERS2.pdf.

Couper, D., Whitman, C., Smith Sloan, K., Marottoli, R., Morgan, H., and Smolski, S. (1999). At the Crossroads: A Guide to Alzheimer's Disease, Dementia and Driving. The Hartford Financial Services Group, Inc., MIT Age Lab and Connecticut Community Care, Inc.

Cummings, J. (2004, July). Alzheimer's Disease, *New England Journal of Medicine*, Volume 351:56–67 July 1, 2004 Number 1.

Dellinger, A., Langlois, J., and Li, G. (2002). Fatal Crashes among Older Drivers: Decomposition of Rates into Contributing Factors. *Am. J. Epidemiol.*, Feb. 155: 234–241.

Dennis, L. (Nov–Jan, 2001). Perspectives—A Newsletter for Individuals with Alzheimer's or a Related Disorder, [6, (2), pp.1–2].

Elkins, D. (1999) Spirituality. *Psychology Today* Sept/Oct 99. (Document ID: 414) Retrieved on June 2, 2004 from http://cms.psychologytoday.com/articles/pto-19990901-000036.html.

Faison, K.J., Faria, S.H., and Frank, D. (1999). Caregivers of chronically ill elderly: Perceived burden. *J. Community Health Nurse.* 1999 Winter;16 (4):243–53.

Family Caregivers on the Job: Moving Beyond ADLS and IADLs. *Generations–Journal of the American Society on Aging*, V. XXVI, No. 4. Families USA (2004). Medicare Prescription Drug Discount Card. Testimony, Ronald F. Pollack, Executive Director Before the Subcommittee on Health Committee on Energy and Commerce, U.S. House of Representatives, May 20, 2004. http://www.familiesusa.org.

Geyer, J.A., Ragland, D.R. Vehicle Occupancy and Crash Risk. Papaer UCB TSCRR200416, (2004). Institute of Transportation studies U.C. Berkley Traffic Safety Center. Abstract 5031.0.Paper presented at American Public Health Association 131st Annual Meeting, San Francisco. Presented Nov. 19, 2003.

Giltay, E.J. (2004, November). Study of Elderly Shows Optimists Have Lower Risk of Death. *Arch. Gen. Psychiatry* (one of the *JAMA* journals) Psychiatric Center GGZ Delfland, Delft, the Netherlands.

Glaser, J-K., Glaser, R. (2003). Chronic stress and age-related increases in the proinflammatory cytokine IL-6, Proceedings of the National Academy of Sciences, June 30, 2003.

Kiecolt-Glaser, J.K., Preacher, K.J., MacCallum, R.C., Atkinson, C., Malarkey, W.B., and Glaser, R. Chronic stress and age-related increases in the proinflammatory cytokine IL-6. Proceedings of the National Academy of Sciences (NAS) 100: 9090-9095; published online before print as 10.1073/pnas.1531903100 www.pnas.org/cgi/content/abstract/100/15/9090.

Gross, D., Raetzman, S., and Schondelmeyer, S.W. (2005). Trends in Manufacturer Prices of Prescription Drugs Used by Older Americans. AARP Studies, http://www.aarp.org/research.

The Hartford (2000). At the Crossroads: A Guide to Alzheimer's Disease, Dementia and Driving. [Brochure]. Hartford, CT. Retrieved June, 2003 from http://www.thehartford.com/alzheimers/105013final.pdf.

Jacobs, B. (2004). What Can I Do? *Take Care!* Vol. 13, No. 2, p. 15–16.

Janke, M.K. (1994). Age Related Disabilities That May Impair Driving and Their Assessment. California Department of Motor Vehicles. National Center for Injury Prevention and Control Synthesis of Human Factors Research on Older Drivers and Highway Safety Vol. I: Older Driver Research Synthesis. http://www.fhwa.dot.gov/tfhrc/safety/pubs/97094/97094.PDF.

Koenig Coste, J. (2004). *Learning to Speak Alzheimer's*, Houghton Mifflin Company, New York.

Levine, C., Reinhard, S.C., Friss Feinberg, L., Albert, S., and Hart, A. (2003–2004, Winter). Family Caregivers on the Job: Moving Beyond ADLS and IADLs., *Generations-J. Am. Society on Aging*, V. XXVI, No. 4.

Lipsitz, L. (2003, October 12). Where Are the Geriatricians? *Boston Globe*. Retrieved April 1, 2005, http://www.boston.com/news/globe.

Lindquist, L. and Golub, R. (2004) Cruise Ship Care: A Proposed Alternative to Assisted Living Facilities. *J. Am. Geriatrics Soc.* 52 (11), 1951–1954. doi: 10.1111/j.1532–5415.2004.52525.x Nov. 2004.

Louis Harris and Associates (1997). Pain and the Older American Survey. Study No. 628200. 6. The Management of Persistent Pain in Older Persons. AGS Panel on Persistent Pain in Older Persons. JAGS 50:S205-S224, 2002 American Geriatrics Society.

Lustbader, W. and Hooyman, N. (1994). Taking Care of Aging Family Members: A Practical Guide. (Rev. ed.) New York: *The Free Press*.

U.S. Dept. Health and Human Services, National Strategy for Suicide Prevention, www.mentalhealth.org.

Meta-Analysis: High-Dosage Vitamin E Supplementation May Increase All-Cause Mortality. *Ann. Intern. Med.* 4 January 2005, Volume 142, No. 1, pp. 37–46.

MetLife Mature Market Institute (2003). The MetLife Study of Sons at Work: Balancing Employment and Eldercare.

McClosky, A. (2000). Cost Overdose: Growth in Drug Spending. for the Elderly, 1992–2010. Families USA Publication No. 00-107. 2000 by Families USA Foundation. http://www.familiesusa.org.

Miller III, E., Pastor-Barriuso, R., Dalal, D., Riemersma, R., and Appel, L. (2004).

Mittelman, M.S., Roth, D.L., Coon, D.W., and Haley, W.E. (2004 ). Sustained Benefit of Supportive Intervention for Depression Symptoms in Caregivers of Patients with Alzheimer's Disease. *Am. J. Psychiatry*; 161:1–7.

Mockus Parks, S. and Novielli, K.D. (2000). A Practical Guide to Caring for Caregivers. American Academy of Family Physicians. http://www.aafp.org.

Morris, M.C., et al. (2002). Dietary Intake of Antioxidant Nutrients and the Risk of Incident Alzheimer Disease. *JAMA*, 287: 3230–3237.

National Advisory Council for Long Term Care Insurance (2005). Fighting Over the Care of Aging Parents -More Siblings Clashing Over Money and Control Retrieved May 31, 2005 from http://www.genpolicy.com/initiatives/fighting_over_aging_parents.html.

National Center on Elder Abuse (2003). Major Types of Elder Abuse: The Basics. Retrieved June 1, 2005, from www.elderabusecenter.org.

National Center for Injury Prevention and Control (NCIPC). Older Adult Drivers: Fact Sheet. (NHTSA 2003) Retrieved Nov. 24, 2004 from www.cdc.gov/ncipc/factsheets/older.hm.

National Council on the Aging (August 2004). Funding Care with Reverse Mortgages.

The National Council on the Aging (NCOA) and The Pew Charitable Trusts. (1997) Nearly 7 Million Long-Distance Caregivers Make Work and Personal Sacrifices. Retrieved March 26, 2005 from http://www.ncoa.org.

National Family Caregivers Association (NFCA) (1998). Caregiving Across the Life Cycle. http://www.nfcacares.org/who/caregiving_survey.cfm.

National Family Caregivers Association. (2000, Oct) Caregiver Survey-2000, Kensington, MD, Retrieved from May 5, 2005 from www.the familycaregiver.org/who/2000_survey.cfm.

Pieters-Hawke, S. and Flynn, H. (2004). *Hazel's Journey: A Personal Experience of Alzheimer's.* Pan MacMillan Australia.

Nielsen//NetRatings. (2003). Senior citizens lead Internet growth, according to the Nielsen//net ratings. Retrieved on May 4, 2004 from http://www.netratings.com/pr/pr_031120.pdf.

O'Neill, G. and Barry, P. (2002). Training Physicians in Geriatric Care: Responding to Critical Need. Public Policy and Aging Report. p. 21 Volume 13, No. 2. http://www.agingsociety.org/agingsociety.

Palley, R. (1998). *Unlikely Passages.* New York: Sheridan House Inc.

Pandya, S. (2005). Caregiving: Caregiving in the United States Research Report. AARP Public Policy Institute. Retrieved June 14, 2005 from http://www.aarp.org/research/housing-obility/caregiving/Articles/fs111_caregiving.html.

Peters, M., Simmons, H. (2001). The Rest of Living. In Simmons, H. and Wilson, J. *Soulful Aging: Ministry Through the Ages of Adulthood.* P133. Macon, Georgia: Smyth and Helwys Publishing, Inc.

Rekate, H. (2004). Saved From Senility, Jeff Fager (Executive Producer) 60 Minutes. New York: CBS. www.cbsnews.com/stories/2004/10/04/6011/main647205.shtml.

Sano, M., et al. (1997). A Controlled Trial of Selegiline, Alpha-Tocopherol, or Both as Treatment for Alzheimer's Disease, *N. Eng. J. Med.* 336, no. 17: 1216–22.

Schorr, M. (2003). Elderly Drivers May Be Safer With a "Co-pilot" 11/20/03. [Medscape Medical News] APHA 131st Annual Meeting: Abstract 5031.0. Presented Nov. 19, 2003.

Schlossberg, N., Waters, E., and Goodman, J. (1995). *Counseling Adults in Transition: Linking Practice With Theory,* 2nd ed., Springer Publishing Company.

SeniorNet, (2002). Seniors online increase. Retrieved Dec. 15, 2002 from http://www.seniorjournal.com/NEWS/SeniorStats/3-02-04SnrsOnline.

Simmons, H.E. and M.A. Goldberg (2003). Charting the Cost of Inaction. National Coalition on Health Care.

Straight, A. and McLarty Jackson, A. (1999). Older Drivers: Fact Sheet. AARP Public Policy Institute. Retrieved Nov. 24, 2004 from www.cdc.gov/ncipc/factsheets/older.htm.

Stucki, B.R. Ph.D. (January 2005). Use Your Home to Stay at Home. Expanding the use of reverse mortages for long term care: A blueprint for action. National Council on the Aging, Washington, D.C.

Yungblut, J. (2001) Dying. In Simmons, H. and Wilson, J. *Soulful Aging: Ministry Through the Ages of Adulthood.* P166. Macon, Georgia: Smyth and Helwys Publishing, Inc.

Yungblut, J. (2001) Ready or Not. In Simmons, H. and Wilson, J. *Soulful Aging: Ministry Through the Ages of Adulthood.* P54. Macon, Georgia:Smyth and Helwys Publishing, Inc.

# Index

*We hope you've enjoyed*

# *Navigating the Journey of Aging Parents: What Care Receivers Want*

*We are interested in your comments.*

*Please contact*
**Cheryl Kuba**
*with your comments, questions, and suggestions at*

## Aging Parent Solutions, LLC
Chicago, IL

Cheryl@agingparentsolutions.com
773-327-2988